EXTREME
HEALING

"This book shows how you, someone with chronic health challenges, can reclaim your health and reframe your struggles. As a Cancer Exercise Specialist who has worked with hundreds of survivors, I know the positive impact exercise has on a patient's recovery. Mari's unique life experience as a person with type 1 diabetes and a three-time survivor of cancer makes her a perfect guide for your endurance journey. You will be amazed at the insights Mari offers you in this book."

CATHY SKINNER, CEO, The Art of Well and NXgenPort

"Mari's superpower is her vulnerability and resilience. In this book, she shares the most painful moments of her life threaded together by her pursuit of feeling and believing she is an athlete. Some sentences brought tears to my eyes while others are overwhelmingly inspiring, leaving her readers in awe.

"I recommend this book to anyone who's struggled, who's felt pain, who's wanted to accomplish something but felt unsure. Mari's story will inspire you to believe in yourself and keep working toward your goals."

GINGER VIEIRA, author of *Exercise with Type 1 Diabetes*

"I met Mari at one of her challenge points ten years ago, and I have watched her live the lessons in this book. It is a personal guide, adaptable to athletes of all levels and many different types of health challenges. She will show you a path of success."

REBECCA MATTISON, MD, endocrinologist

"Mari's decades of living with type 1 diabetes and surviving cancer three times, alongside being a successful endurance athlete, provide a powerful recipe for inspiration and instruction for any journey you embark on. Mari shares so much of herself and sets you up with a headstart on your path. Learn how to take charge and accomplish the goals of your dreams by reading this book today! I could not have accomplished *two* 100-mile bike rides and a half-marathon without her help, and I am forever grateful!"

SCOTT K. JOHNSON, blogger, speaker, writer, advocate;
Dx T1D April 26, 1980

"You can put your health in Mari Ruddy's capable hands. . . . Mari's influence, and what I see as magic, comes from how seriously she takes her role as a health promoter and role model. Every single time I follow Mari's thinking and perspective, I benefit. . . . Mari Ruddy helps people put structures in place that make thriving not only possible but likely, even on a bad day. . . .

"I encourage anyone looking for help taking full charge of their health to invest your time in absorbing the wisdom in *Extreme Healing*. You are worth it, and I promise you won't regret it."

LINDA BRANDT, MPH, renegade community builder,
health promotion specialist

"Mari is an athlete who has been able to utilize the tools to endure not only long-distance races but also type 1 diabetes and three rounds of cancer. Her book will help guide you through your own chronic health challenges by taking the driver's seat to successfully steer through even unexpected turns in your life."

JOCELIN HUANG, MD, medical oncologist

"Mari is an athlete first and a person with type 1 diabetes and a three-time survivor of cancer second. . . . I've known Mari for more than ten years, and you will not be disappointed in the guidance Mari offers you in this book."

MANNY HERNANDEZ, @askmanny, diabetes advocate,
living with diabetes since October 2002

"Mari embodies the lessons she teaches in her book as an athlete and friend everyday. I see the curiosity, commitment and fun that Mari has by choosing to pursue her goals with her whole self, reaching out for help when she needs it and bringing others along for the ride. She has a ride to take you on in her book, *Extreme Healing*, that will show you the path to becoming an athlete, overcomer, and lifelong learner."

DANIEL DOCHERTY, two-time US Olympic Trials Marathon qualifier,
elite athlete, coach, and program director

EXTREME HEALING

EXTREME HEALING

RECLAIM YOUR LIFE
✚ LEARN TO LOVE
YOUR BODY

MARI RUDDY

Published by

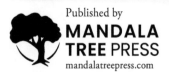

MANDALA TREE PRESS
mandalatreepress.com

Paperback ISBN: 9781954801585
Hardcover ISBN: 9781954801608
eBook ISBN: 9781954801615

HEA007000   HEALTH & FITNESS / Exercise / General
SEL021000   SELF-HELP / Motivational & Inspirational
HEA039050   HEALTH & FITNESS / Diseases & Conditions / Diabetes

Cover design and typesetting by Kaitlin Barwick
Edited by Deborah Spencer
Photos by Amy Anderson

mariruddy.com

To all the athletes I've met and
all of you that I one day will meet.
You all inspire me.

Remember, athletic talent is
best measured by your internal gauge.
Keep moving your body.
You're worth it.

CONTENTS

CONTENTS

FOREWORD

THE TWO GREATEST MOTIVATORS IN LIFE ARE FEAR AND desire. Author and athlete Mari Ruddy's book, *Extreme Healing*, shares both of these motivators wrapped with personal stories that fuse the intimate and sometimes troubling challenges with the positive successes in her life's journey. This personal and revealing book intertwines personal experiences with cancer, friendships, diabetes, suicide, childhood trauma, bankruptcy, family stress, and athletic challenges. All of these real-life experiences are delivered to you from her heart and her life's path.

Through all that life has thrown at Mari in the past five decades, of the two motivators of fear and desire she has experienced, participation in athletic and fitness activities has supported her travels to find a place she sought: a life of happiness. With her persistence and cheerful attitude, she was able to fuse the courage and willingness to try new and difficult activities—mental, emotional, and physical—that at one time seemed beyond her ability and capacity. She did it. She found her happy place.

Mari Ruddy provides you with more than just insights into an American woman's life challenges today; she also brings the tools to overcome those really tough times and experience the outcomes—some good and some bad. But with honesty and clarity, she puts them together in a compelling story of how she devised plans and solutions, and how she developed a map to change the downward spiral into upward achievements.

In this powerfully moving book, she writes, "As I reflect on the challenges of my life—the sexual abuse, the diabetes, the three rounds of cancer, the attachment disorder, the suicide attempts, the estrangement from my biological family, the challenges I have had with trusting friendships—all of it reminds me that despite these challenges, I chose it. I have learned from all of these horrible experiences."

If you are looking for a touchstone in your life, if you are ready for a different life trajectory, if embracing fitness and health is one of your life's goals, then read this work—it's just that great.

SALLY EDWARDS, MA

Author, Professional Triathlete, Techpreneur, and Founder of Heart Zones and Fleet Feet. Sacramento, California. (October 5, 2022)

INTRODUCTION

SET THE STAGE

"Endurance is one of the most difficult
disciplines, but it is to the one who
endures that the final victory comes."

—*BUDDHA*

"YOU ARE ON THE FAST TRACK TO DEATH. YOU ARE IN TER-rible health. Your diabetes is out of control. You had better do something different, or you have very little time left," my doctor said in her office that Tuesday morning. On my drive home, I had to pull over to avoid being in a car accident due to the tears streaming down my face. Sitting in my car, I let the sobs wrack my body.

Fear coursed through me, landing in my belly with a clench every time I tried to go for a run or ride my bike for longer than a few blocks. The sexual abuse I survived as a child taught me to avoid feeling my body and resulted in a paralyz-ing fear of exercising. The fear kept me reading on the couch and eating bags of chips. I was tired most of the time, and I often and easily got sick. I had lived almost half my life with poorly managed diabetes, largely due to my fear of exercising. I had also survived three exhausting rounds of breast cancer

1

and two desperate suicide attempts. I wanted to change, but I wasn't sure how.

If you've ever gone through the devastating impact of a health diagnosis, this book is for you. Perhaps you too don't know how to change your health for the better. I can completely relate. It wasn't until I found the endurance sports of triathlon (cycling, running, swimming), and cross-country skiing that I felt like I had found hope. In this book, I share with you how I found my way, and how you too can find your way.

There are three reasons I like endurance sports. First, I live with a chronic health condition—type 1 diabetes. Second, I have thrice survived breast cancer. And third, going back even further to my childhood, I spent eleven years in fear of family members and caregivers who sexually abused me. These three reasons, and a few others I will share, are why endurance sports have saved my life over and over.

There have been many days that I felt like I was simply enduring. I woke up in the morning, looking ahead to the day, not knowing if I would be safe, not knowing if my health would hold up. That forced me to dig deep inside myself for strength and courage to just get out of bed and embrace the day.

Now, as an endurance athlete, when I'm out cycling, running, swimming, or cross-country skiing and I hit a crippling level of pain, it reminds me of the moments I hit when my blood sugar isn't in range. It reminds me of the five chemotherapy sessions or the thirty-six radiation treatments I endured. It reminds me of the frightening betrayal I felt when someone who was supposed to protect me overstepped boundaries and took advantage of my young body. In those moments of remembering, I tell myself that I survived all those gigantic, seemingly insurmountable challenges, and I am actually choosing to be out there running, cycling, swimming, or cross-country skiing. I realize I *love* these sports! That brings a smile to my face, and I discover yet another level of strength to move into and beyond the crippling pain.

To endure is to remain in existence, to last, or to suffer patiently. Endurance sports test your ability to do so over long distances. Along with my preferred cycling, running, swimming, and cross-country skiing, there's inline skating, rowing, mountain biking, race walking, trail running, paddling, and even more sports. The focus in endurance sports is on how you show up with the distance, time, and physical and mental pain, and whether you complete the event you set out to do. Very rarely is the emphasis on how fast you go or how your performance compares to that of other athletes competing. "Slowly and surely" wins the race every time, and the best part is that in most endurance events *everyone* gets a medal for finishing.

For those of us who agonize about our health conditions, weight, or age, endurance athletics offers a beautiful parallel. By that, I mean it doesn't do much good to compare yourself to others in either case. I learned the hard way that comparing myself to others gets me exactly nothing. I'm not fast and that's okay. In fact, when my competitive side creeps out (which it does) and I start comparing myself to the runners or cyclists who are going twice as fast as I am, I've thankfully learned instead to tune into what is happening in my body at that moment.

What does matter is how you are managing your health, weight, or age. Living with diabetes or cancer or asthma or any other chronic health condition is *not* a sprint. It's much more like a 100-mile bike ride or a marathon in that it requires digging deeply inside yourself and finding the strength and courage to keep showing up in the face of setbacks, complications, and surprises.

Discovering endurance athletics completely enhanced my life for the better. It helped me safely and strongly reclaim my body after the sexual abuse forced me out of it. It helped me discover lifesaving ways to live with my diabetes and cancer. Best of all, it connected me to circles of inspiring people who love living life as healthfully as they can. I offer this book as a catalyst as you too discover the power of endurance sports to guide you through whatever life and health challenges you are facing.

The book is organized into thirteen chapters, each one building on the last. I start with guiding you to claim the identity of an athlete. Then we will discuss health challenges, focusing on what you go through when you get a chronic health diagnosis, like diabetes or cancer. We will explore the challenges that arise as we strive for better health, and how to overcome these challenges. Moving forward, we explore the fear and obstacles that get in the way of becoming active, since fear and obstacles can stop us from taking action. You are worth figuring out the fear and overcoming the obstacles. We then dive into the power of signing up for a race or event, and how that invites you to gather your team around you to prepare for the event you signed up to do. To keep it fun and engaging, we look at what to wear and why having good athletic clothing makes a positive difference in your performance. You need some gear to be a success, so we'll get into how to find the right gear. Taking things deeper, we explore how to eat like an athlete and how to optimize sleep and recovery, things that will make a positive difference in your health and well-being overall. Which leads to exploring training plans and race plans that will prepare you for the event you will do. Then we discuss how to manage the post-race letdown that many athletes experience. Knowing that might happen will help you frame and deal when or if that arises. Finally, we talk about how to continue to find the energy and focus to be a year-round endurance athlete, no matter your age or health challenges. Then in chapter thirteen, I tie it all together. Reminding you of your strength, power, and endurance ability to make yourself an endurance athlete. To wrap up the book (in the event you're curious), in the bonus chapter I tell the story of how and why I created the Red Rider Program, which is used at The American Diabetes Association Tour de Cure events.

Along the way you will get to know my story, how I battled, struggled, and found my way by going inward. And how, in the process, I found joy in my body. My hope is that you too will find your courage to regain your health, wellness, and athletic self. You are worth it.

I'm glad you are here on this adventure with me!

MARI RUDDY

CHAPTER 1

BELIEF

I AM AN ATHLETE

"The basic difference between an ordinary
man or woman and a warrior is that a warrior
takes everything as a challenge, while an
ordinary man or woman takes everything
either as a blessing or a curse."

—*CARLOS CASTANEDA*

MY ASSUMPTION IS THAT IF YOU ARE HOLDING THIS BOOK
in your hands, you want to become an athlete. Maybe you
already are an athlete and were diagnosed with a health
condition or had your life similarly disrupted. Perhaps your
weight is more than you want it to be, or you realize you're
older than you'd like. You want to know you aren't alone, and
you seek reassurance that you can still be an athlete even with
the challenges you face.

I'm assuming a few other things too. I assume you're smart
and that no matter where you are right now, you can figure this
out. I've worked in schools where the teachers used a system
called the Solution Focused Approach[1] when interacting with
high-risk youth. The approach assumes that everyone has expe-
rienced success in some area of life and, when facing a new

challenge, can extrapolate the skills and behaviors from that past success to apply them to a new challenge.

This approach deeply resonates with me because, in my life, it has worked—over and over again. And this is what I assume about you. You've had success somewhere in your life and you can draw upon it as you dive into becoming an athlete. Said another way: you got this. As you read this book, keep reminding yourself of your successes. Just like how you succeeded in those areas, you can also succeed at being an athlete. As of right now, you *are* an athlete. Declare it to be true.

You might have an argument with this. How can just saying you're an athlete make you one? Well, you have to start somewhere, and sometimes you just have to try on a new self-image and declare it to be true, even if it's just to get yourself to start.

In my case, I didn't even like to exercise and had every reason in the world to avoid it. I have lived with type 1 diabetes since I was sixteen years old. I survived breast cancer three times. I have exercise-induced asthma. I am a childhood sexual abuse survivor who could only make peace with what had happened to me by avoiding living "in" my body and tuning out its messages. Starting when I was twelve years old, I thought I was fat, and it took a long time to make peace with the size of my body. Never a skinny Minnie, I've experimented with practically every sort of diet, and my exercise prior to age thirty consisted of having five different gym memberships in seven years. I made it inside the gym nine times. I, obviously, had to do something differently. Additionally, I attempted suicide shortly after my initial diabetes diagnosis when I was a teenager and then again twice when I was an adult. Ironically, I don't suffer from depression, unusual for someone who attempts suicide multiple times in their life. Instead, what I suffer from is PTSD from the intense traumas I've survived in my life. Suicide was an attempt to escape the unbearable pain of feeling like I didn't belong anywhere and not knowing who I was and not feeling successful at anything I attempted to accomplish.

I applied the Solution Focused Approach to myself. I had been both a high school principal and a coach to high-powered executives, helping them be more successful. The motivator I was in those roles, those worlds, saw clearly that success begins with what you think of yourself. I needed to apply that notion to myself. I strongly encourage you to try this too. Think about your own life and remember in particular all the accomplishments and successes you've had. Breathe into your own successful reality. Keep those top of mind as we move into this next step.

Declaring myself an athlete didn't mean I would become one, but I felt different after saying it. It was as if I were there on the starting line instead of already behind and feeling like a slug. I decided to go with it. I knew the simpler I kept it, the more likely I would be to actualize it. My declaration was

I am an athlete.

Declaring myself an athlete was like cleaning windows. Growing up in Minnesota, we had to change out the summertime screens for storm windows every fall in preparation for winter. My mom had a particular passion for clean windows and enlisted my siblings and me to make the job of cleaning the eighteen-some windows a little easier. The adage "many hands make light work" was one of her favorites. Minnesota winters are bleak, and Mom wanted every drop of sunshine and light to make it into the house. At the time, it just seemed like another chore she dreamed up to keep us out of trouble. Now, looking back, I am grateful for learning the value of a sparkling clean window through which to see the world. Just like when we wiped those dirty windows clean, I enjoy when life comes into sharp focus, as it does when you declare yourself to be an athlete with clear intention.

I needed to wipe off my inactive body and see the potential for movement underneath. Although uncomfortable at first, I discovered that I liked this new self-image. It felt powerful inside to say, "I am an athlete." I started viewing the world through this new, bright, clear lens and found myself wondering, "What would an athlete do now?" "What would an athlete eat?" "Do athletes keep track of that?"

WHAT IS AN ATHLETE?

Everyone has a different idea of what being an athlete means. My sister, who, at the time, had completed seven marathons, told me she wasn't an athlete because she wasn't very good at sports. Her husband was an athlete, she said, because he was a gifted soccer player and had grace and technical skill. A lot of people think this way—that you have to be good at a sport to call yourself an athlete.

Not me. If you are human and can move your body, you are an athlete. Sure, it's a broad definition, but what a powerful way to define yourself. I went on to not only become an athlete but also (by my late-thirties) an endurance athlete, which means I do sports that involve doing aerobic exercise for longer than ninety minutes. When I started, I didn't know that going on long hikes or bike rides was considered "endurance." I just knew I liked them. I enjoyed seeing how far I could go while still having fun.

Finding my athletic self, discovering how much freedom and satisfaction I gained when I could finally be *in* my body, transformed my daily reality. The beautiful magic all started when I changed my mind and declared myself an athlete.

Please. Start with changing your mind.

The first person who helped me consider the possibility of calling myself an athlete was my dear friend and former romantic partner Chris Klebl. Chris and I met at a Holotropic Breathwork®2 and meditation retreat in 1999 in Joshua Tree, California. Chris was born in Germany to an American mother and an Austrian father. At an early age, he learned to ski and snowboard in the Alps. He spoke German and English, but when he was fifteen and enrolled at an East Coast boarding school in the United States, he realized his knowledge of American pop culture and teenage humor wasn't up to speed. He was grateful for his skiing and snowboarding skills because being athletic helped level the teenage playing field.

After college, Chris moved to Colorado and found a group of snowboarding friends. Chris and his pals were adventurous, often jumping off cliffs and finding ungroomed trails to snowboard. One day, Chris was following his friends off a big jump (about thirty-five feet). Mid-air, he knew something was wrong. His next memory was lying in the snow and feeling the cold snow up his jacket. He couldn't move. The rescue team found him and brought down the mountain. He was then airlifted to Craig Hospital in Denver. At age twenty-three, Chris had broken his spinal cord. He could no longer walk or feel his legs. For several years, Chris's attention was focused on navigating his new, more difficult life. He slowly and surely began to lift weights, wanting to find his athlete self again.

I met Chris at that meditation retreat with teachers Jack Kornfield and Stanislav Grof.[3] I was struck by how tall he sat. His posture was the straightest in the room. I could feel his athletic prowess, even though it was dormant. Chris moved from Kauai to live with me in Santa Cruz, California. Within a few months of moving to Santa Cruz, Chris decided he wanted to start hand cycling, and he asked his parents to help buy him one. Six weeks after he got this amazing bike, he decided he wanted to enter some races. He recruited me to help him train. Chris was an excellent example to me of the power of deciding on a path and believing in yourself.

STARTING TO RIDE

I got my old, green hybrid bike out of the shed, inflated the tires, and polished it up. Chris and I would go for rides that would last an hour, then longer. The rides got difficult on that old hybrid bike. Chris and I made a plan. After 100 rides on that old green hybrid, I could get a new road bike. I kept a tally of every ride I did. Slowly but surely, I got closer to 100. On the journey, I went with Chris to his first races. I saw amputees and other paraplegic athletes and the question I asked myself was, "These folks can't walk and here they are racing. What's my issue? I can walk. I just have diabetes."

Perspective makes a big difference. Diabetes isn't small potatoes, but compared to not having a limb, it made me realize maybe I could figure it out. Little by little, I realized I could race. When I got to 100 rides on the old hybrid, Chris went with me to get a new road bike. He insisted that I ride at least five bikes. I was so nervous riding those bikes. I wasn't used to riding a road bike; I had gotten comfortable on that old hybrid bike. Chris talked me through my nerves, reminding me that I had earned a shiny new bike. I had saved up money and now was the time to get a bike to match my new level of fitness. I got a steel bike with a carbon fiber fork. It was an entry-level racing bike, a LeMond Zurich. To this day, I still own that bike, and I love it as dearly as the day I bought it.

STARTING TO RACE

Chris convinced me to sign up for a women's racing clinic. I met Nicole Freedman, the coach. She rode next to me during much of the clinic, encouraging me, pushing me to go harder. Much to my surprise, Nicole immediately saw something in me. She liked my persistence, my cheerful attitude, and my willingness to try all the drills she put before us. She noticed that I was attentive to my diabetes needs, but not demanding about them. She sensed, even before I did, that I had a quiet physical confidence.

In the meantime, Chris kept racing too. He got in touch with the coaching staff of the US Paralympic Cycling Team. He kept getting better and better. When we rode together, he would draft behind me. He'd yell at me to keep cycling in perfect circles. If I needed to stop because of my diabetes, it was no big deal for Chris. We'd stop and take care of whatever it was. This calm, focused way of dealing with the what-seemed-to-me-constant challenge of diabetes was just another moment in life to Chris. I found myself breathing more deeply and beginning to trust this new approach to life's challenges.

From Chris, I learned a new way to be with my diabetes. I found myself calmer and more confident.

Then we moved to Colorado. Chris was unsatisfied with his progress with hand cycling, so he got the Paralympic cycling coach to take him cross-country sit skiing. He knew that since he'd loved snowboarding, he would likely love cross-country skiing. Within a short time, Chris was winning races and he was passionate about every aspect of the sport, including developing designs for a new bucket to sit in. Soon, he traded in his hand cycle for a roller board on which he could mount his sit ski frame and, with different poles, push himself in a similar manner over dry land and pavement. He figured out a way to create a pull-up system that built up the muscles in his abs, shoulders, and arms. He was bound and determined to make progress in sit skiing.

ATHLETES KEEP RECORDS OF EVERYTHING

I learned about athlete recordkeeping from Chris. He logged everything. The weather conditions when he trained. How much sleep he got. How much he ate. Exactly what terrain he trained on and for how long. This made diabetes recordkeeping look like child's play. People with diabetes are encouraged to keep track of their daily medications, the exact carbohydrates, all food eaten and at what time, and their level of blood glucose as tested throughout the day and night. It's a lot of recordkeeping. Again, perspective helps frame things.

Chris developed training plans based on Olympic cross-country skiers, able-bodied ones, on the teams in Scandinavia and Russia. He desperately wanted a good coach. He met one when he was in New Zealand at the Snow Farm where cross-country skiers from all over the world go to train in August. The coach was from Canada.

After the 2010 Olympics in Vancouver, British Columbia (in which Chris competed as a US Paralympic sit skier), Chris decided it was time to go ski with the Canadian coach. This meant it was time to look into becoming a Canadian citizen. He moved to Canmore, Alberta, Canada, home of some of the best cross-country skiing in the world. And he kept skiing fast. He was very happy to have found teammates he liked, ski techs who understood his meticulous passion for finding the correct wax, and a coach who could help him reach his peak.

In February 2014, Chris flew to Sochi, Russia, for the Paralympics (which are held at the same venue as the Olympics) two weeks later. He skied in several races. Then it was the 10K race. Much to everyone's surprise but his, he won. He got the gold medal. An Olympic gold. Who knows what's possible for you? Maybe you will win a race. Maybe you will go to the Olympics. Maybe you'll improve your health. Maybe you'll simply find a lifelong joy in endurance athletics. It all begins with believing you are an athlete.

DECLARE YOUR IDENTITY

The power of declaring an identity for yourself, even before it's 100 percent true, may seem silly. I know that early on using the term "athlete" for myself felt ridiculous. I just kept breathing into it and each exercise session I did was a tiny bit of evidence that I was on my way. I've had a lot of setbacks in my life and have gotten out of fitness shape many times. Getting out of shape and then deciding to get back in fitness shape requires fortitude and strength and even a bit of courage. What helps me the most is starting each recommitment to getting my body and mind back in good fitness by declaring myself an athlete. It's so simple and so effective. Then before each exercise session (before I start running, biking, swimming, or cross-country skiing), I take thirty seconds to a minute to take a deep breath or two and say to myself, "I am an athlete. Athletes feel their bodies. Athletes train. I am doing what an athlete does. Remember, Mari, you are an athlete." It's powerful *and* magical.

VISION BOARDS

Early in starting TeamWILD Athletics LLC, I knew that taking a moment to envision yourself as an athlete was essential. I knew this because it took me a while to state that I was an athlete and then to also say it aloud to people. Vision boards are something I've done for many years.

On the first night of TeamWILD camps, we had everyone make a vision board declaring themselves an athlete. I reached out to my network of triathlon friends and gathered as many bicycling, running, swimming, and triathlon magazines as I could find. We would then begin camp by creating a collage of images and words that declared ourselves as athletes. We would start imagining ourselves as athletes as we cut out pictures and words in different fonts. As people used scissors and glue sticks, they would talk about themselves as athletes. We found ourselves sharing our hesitations and our excitement for camp. After a few hours of cutting and pasting, we went around the room and each of us shared our board and how we were feeling about embracing the title "athlete."

I was the director of the camp, and I too made a vision board at the start of every camp. Over the years we held five CampWILDs, and I made five vision boards declaring myself an athlete. Each time I made one, I felt more sure of myself using that moniker. The cringing and hesitation I felt using the word "athlete" to describe myself got a bit easier as time went by. I've realized how helpful and transformative it is to simply begin with the desired outcome in mind. I wasn't comfortable with calling myself an athlete, but I kept doing it anyway. My hope was that eventually it would become comfortable. That is what finally happened. Believe in yourself and it will happen for you too.

TRY THIS

Step one is to change your mind and your belief system. Step two is to take action. To help with this process, in each chapter, I will have an action item or two for you to do to help move you along on the path to becoming an endurance athlete.

Journal

Please find a notebook to dedicate for use as you read this book. Today, write "I am an athlete" five times. In a few sentences, describe how it feels to make that declaration. Let yourself feel all the emotions of what it is like to call yourself an athlete.

Action

Make a vision board of yourself as an athlete. This will help you create and hold onto the image of yourself as an athlete.

Be sure to put your vision board somewhere where you will see it every day.

Notes

1. Insoo Kim Berg, "What is the Solution Focused Approach?", Solutions Centre, 2004, https://www.solutions-centre.org/what-is-the-solution-focused-approach.
2. "About Holotropic Breathwork," GROF Transpersonal Training, http://www.holotropic.com/holotropic-breathwork/about-holotropic-breathwork.
3. "Dr. Stanislav Grof," https://www.stangrof.com.

Resources

Vision Boards: https://www.betterup.com/blog/how-to-create-vision-board

CHAPTER 2

HEALTH CONCERNS

BE AN ATHLETE AFTER AND THROUGH DIAGNOSIS

"Knowing others is intelligence; knowing yourself is true wisdom. Mastering others is strength; mastering yourself is true power."

—*LAO TZU*, TAO TE CHING

"WHO AM I?"

This is a question I've been asking myself since I was a child. In fact, I've been searching for myself my entire life. Every day in kindergarten, I walked to the bus stop through all types of small-town Minnesota weather with a huge coat box full of options for show-and-tell. I wanted to be able to jump in to fill any show-and-tell gaps, as I hoped to be accepted and liked by my teacher and my classmates. My five-year-old self wanted to belong. These days I understand that my young self didn't have a sense of belonging to my family. I remember wondering if I was the same as or different from my classmates and not knowing how to find the answer. I remember the lost and empty feeling inside me most of all.

DIABETES DIAGNOSIS

My quest to know myself took on new depth when, one month after turning sixteen, I was diagnosed with type 1 diabetes. Those of us who live with a chronic health challenge, or have survived a health crisis, remember the day we found out that life as we knew it would no longer be the same.

My date was June 26, 1981. I was sitting on the couch with my dad watching the at-home-test tape that measures glucose in the urine and revealed that my pancreas was no longer working. My kidneys couldn't handle the glucose in my system. That morning, I had gone to a birthday celebration for a high school friend. I had eaten cake, regular soda (not something I usually had access to), and lots of picnic-style lunchtime food such as fruit salad, sandwiches, and chips. In other words, I had eaten countless carbohydrates. I didn't know in 1981 that all those carbohydrates make the blood sugar go high in someone who doesn't make insulin any longer. As I watched the test tape turn a dark color, tears cascading down my face, the life my teenage-self imagined was forever changed. Who was I? And who would I be now? My quest for the answer began in earnest.

IT RUNS IN THE FAMILY

I grew up with a father who had type 1 diabetes, and he chose to blend in most of the time. He didn't announce to the world that he had diabetes. Only those of us who were close to him knew. In part, we knew because of the black and blue marks all over his stomach and legs from the needles he used to inject insulin into his body. My dad was diagnosed in 1966, back in the day when people with diabetes took one or two shots of pork or beef insulin with needles they sharpened with hand-held whetting stones and boiled over the stove to sanitize.

The needles hurt, and they were big, so they often left bruises. We also knew (because there was no blood sugar testing) he often had what is known as hypoglycemic unawareness. Meaning he wouldn't be aware of his blood sugar dropping down to dangerously low levels until he started shaking uncontrollably. My father was 6 feet 4 inches tall and when he started shaking, it took at least two men to hold him still to get glucose into him. As a result, at least once a year the paramedics came to my house to help my dad. Each time, I would stand stiff next to my younger brother and sister, fear coursing through my body. Being the oldest, I attempted to reassure them that Dad would be okay. Each time I wondered if he would die this time. I didn't fully understand what death meant, just that he would be forever gone, and that was terrifying.

Sitting in the den the day we figured out I almost for sure had diabetes also, I understood my father and the perilous, difficult nature of living day-to-day with type 1 diabetes. Suddenly I got the struggle to attempt to balance the injected insulin levels, stress, exercise, and food intake. Facing my own diagnosis, I keenly felt the toll that the continual trauma of living with someone who had type 1 diabetes had taken on me growing up.

A day later, in the doctor's office, getting the official diabetes diagnosis, my world crashed around me. I was afraid and wondered if I would die before even turning twenty. I wondered what low blood sugar would feel like. I prayed I wouldn't cause my loved ones as much distress as my father had caused our family. I wondered how I would navigate daily life. I wondered if I would ever again feel hope.

CHRONIC ILLNESS DIAGNOSIS FOLLOWS GRIEF STAGES

It turns out that I was navigating the stages of grief.[1] Anytime one of us is diagnosed with a chronic illness, we go through these various stages of grief. Not necessarily in a straight line, since we might skip back and forth between the stages. It's even possible to skip some of the stages altogether. You've likely heard of the five stages of grief as outlined by Elizabeth Kubler-Ross. The stages are denial, anger, bargaining, depression, and acceptance.

I'd always marched to my own drummer; therefore, I wasn't surprised that, along with my distress, a glimmer of defiance began to emerge. The defiance was me bargaining. I wondered if maybe, somehow, some way, there was a different way to approach the disease. Maybe this wasn't the end of my life, but a chance to do things differently. I didn't know how or if it was even possible, but something within me yelled just loudly enough that my sixteen-year-old self could hear. It was my Inner Healer[2] introducing itself to me. This is sometimes called the Inner Healing Intelligence. It made itself known right after my diabetes diagnosis. A blessing in disguise.

Upon my own diagnosis, I was rebellious, as is normal for a sixteen-year-old. I chose not to blend in. I announced to everyone that I had diabetes. I became a walking encyclopedia about diabetes. I took the bus to the Minnesota office of the American Diabetes Association, and I became a counselor at Camp Needlepoint, the local camp for children with diabetes.

This desire to not blend in was my way of coping with the difficult challenge of having diabetes myself, after growing up with the constant threat of wondering if diabetes would kill my father. I hoped that alerting people about my diabetes would create more acceptance for those with diabetes, which might have helped my father navigate his disease with more openness and care. I now understand that this public announcement of my diagnosis was another layer of anger and bargaining.

FOUNDATIONAL PRACTICES

Have you heard the voice of *your* Inner Healer? I believe all of us have one within us. Some of us are able to hear this wisdom early and easily. Others of us are never taught or never learn to trust this inner wisdom. I think because I had such an active imagination and I continuously searched to feel a sense of belonging, I learned early to listen to my own inner wisdom, which I believe holds our Inner Healer. This early attention to my Inner Healer was a result of being in a family where I felt disconnected from nearly everyone. I had deep distrust of most of the caregivers in my life, so I learned to tune into my own inner voices. Decisions I made after the diabetes diagnosis laid the foundation for how I would relate to my disease and to my health.

One strategy I adopted was to take full advantage of the new tools available in the diabetes community. I was an early adopter of blood glucose testing versus urine analysis to measure glucose in the system. I moved fairly quickly from one shot a day to two to four to six, and then to an insulin pump. I learned how to count food exchanges using guidelines from the American Dietetic Association and the American Diabetes

Association. Later, I learned how to count carbohydrates and closely match insulin to food intake. My Inner Healer guided me to learn everything I could about my condition.

I kept meticulous records and became obsessed with learning everything from them as well as from science and medicine. I always brought a list of questions to my doctor visits, a practice I still do today. My thirst for knowledge and understanding were my lifelines to hope.

The decision I made at age sixteen to avoid hard exercise had dire consequences. Exercise is a key component of overall good health in general and sound diabetes management in particular. It's not that I completely avoided exercise; but I never pushed my body too hard, having watched how my father experienced low blood sugars more frequently and intensely during or after exercise. In the name of avoiding those frightening lows, I also ran my blood sugars just a bit high by not quite taking enough insulin. Fourteen years after being diagnosed and living with diabetes, the culmination of these choices came to a head.

CONSEQUENCES STRIKE

I was thirty years old and the endocrinologist I was seeing at the time read me the riot act after a key test showed I was squarely in the range of "very poorly managed diabetes and you might die if you don't do something about it soon." My glycosylated hemoglobin test, known as an A1c, was almost 13 percent, which is quite high. An A1c test measures the glucose that has attached to the red blood cells, or hemoglobin, as they form, with the test indicating overall blood sugar management. "If you don't do something soon, you'll be blind, have kidney failure, or have a heart attack," the endocrinologist said, continuing on. "As if those aren't bad enough, you could have complete organ failure resulting in death before you reach the ripe old age of thirty-five."

I left the office and started sobbing. Alone with tears falling down my face, I asked myself, "Who am I?" "How did this happen to me?" and "What can I do about it?" I didn't dwell on the "What did I do to deserve this?" loop, having watched my father make little progress in coming up with any answers to that question. Instead, I opted for questions that could lead to action. Discovering that my A1c was through the roof was an opportunity for me to redefine myself. It was an opportunity to change.

Getting new, difficult information about my chronic health condition thrust me right back into the stages of grief. I was angry and depressed, and I did some bargaining. It took me a little while to get to acceptance. I offer you this information about the stages of grief because it's important to understand the grief stages and know that it is normal to experience grief when your sense of who you are in the world and how you live your life is thrown a curveball. Knowing what you're going through, being able to name it and get appropriate support as you navigate, makes it easier. Even if just a little bit.

At this moment of grief, I was presented with an opportunity to change. As happens when one is presented with such an opportunity, you can choose to transform. At this moment, I had my own transformation to make. I was in a place in my life where I was ready. Perhaps you too are ready. Consider this: The Stages of Change. It helped me.

STAGES OF CHANGE
FOR TRANSFORMATION

The Transtheoretical Model, also known as the Stages of Change, is used by medical practitioners to help assess a patient's readiness to change their behavior in pursuit of better health. Depending on where a patient lands in those stages, the practitioner uses a different approach to help them move toward transformation.

I keep this model in mind in my work as an educator, since it helps guide me in choosing the best strategy to help my students embrace the concepts being studied. A few years into my use of it with others, I realized I could use it on myself, when I don't have a teacher around to help me. I offer it to you to use as you integrate into your life the concepts in this book.

The Stages of Change Described[3]

Pre-contemplation is the stage at which there is no intention in the foreseeable future to change behavior. Many people in this stage are unaware or under-aware of their problems.

I knew before I went to the endocrinologist to get my A1c results that I probably wasn't in peak health, but I didn't know how bad things really were. I was tired most of the time, and I knew I probably should have been exercising. I knew, too, that I should stop under-insulinizing myself, but I didn't have a plan. I didn't even really want to make any changes. Completely unmotivated, I figured I was probably just fine.

Contemplation is the stage in which people are aware that a problem exists and are seriously thinking about overcoming it but have yet to commit to taking action.

I moved from precontemplation to contemplation the day I made the appointment to see the endocrinologist. I hadn't been to see a diabetes specialist in more than a year, and was avoiding taking action, but I was tired of being tired. I had done a series of hypnotherapy sessions. The messages that kept emerging from my body were "Please pay attention" and "Please get some information."

Making the appointment with the endocrinologist was the contemplation stage, since what I was doing was gathering information about my health, but not yet making any changes. I made the appointment with great trepidation, but I did make it. I went in for bloodwork a week before, knowing that the results would give the doctor and me something meaningful to discuss. I'd begun to think that changing something might be a good idea. I wasn't ready to actually make any changes, but I was open to conversation about what might need to change.

Preparation is a stage that combines intention and behavioral criteria. Individuals in this stage have unsuccessfully taken action in the past year but intend to take action within the next month.

I made the shift from contemplation to preparation driving home from the aforementioned appointment. First, I pulled over and cried. This put me back in the stages of grief. I was angry with the endocrinologist. I despaired about my future.

As often happens for me, from the depth of tears emerged the insight that I could apply the skills and knowledge I had from my career as an educator to help with my health. This moved me into acceptance and problem-solving. I spent the rest of the drive home reviewing what I knew from my job as a high school leadership teacher who helped teenagers create meaningful visions for themselves: write a mission statement, set goals, and create task lists to actualize those goals. To my astonishment, I realized I had all of the tools at my fingertips to lower my A1c. By the time I pulled into my driveway, I knew I could do it. Walking in the door, the first thing I did was locate a binder and label it "Mari's Health."

Action is the stage in which individuals modify their behavior, experiences, or environment in order to overcome their problems. Action involves the most overt behavioral changes and requires considerable commitment of time and energy.

My first action item? "Fire my endocrinologist. Find a new doctor who's willing to help me figure this out."

Defiance is a funny thing in the medical field. Some studies have shown[4] that patients who ask a ton of questions and appear less compliant have higher survival rates than those who do everything their doctors tell them to do. I like doctors and am grateful there are people willing to study medicine and devote their lives to helping people. I don't, however, believe that doctors are gods. They are human beings like us who have opinions, make mistakes, and are shaped by their particular life circumstances. Some I click with, and some I don't.

The endocrinologist who gave me the results of my A1c was not an empathetic woman. She frightened me, painting a graphic, horrible picture of the things happening in my body as a result of the excess sugar in my bloodstream. She didn't offer ideas or strategies to change the course I was on, or express any willingness to guide me as I embarked on my journey to wellness. What her approach did, however, was catapult me into action, and for that I will always be grateful.

But fear isn't a sustainable motivator: What I needed and wanted was a teacher.

THE TEACHER SHOWS UP

It was at this point that the right teacher showed up. Her name was Sue Moen, and she was a personal trainer who was willing to work with me and my fears of low blood sugar. She believed I could be an athlete. She was willing to walk the path at my side as I explored becoming one. Sue wasn't rattled by my desire, and need, to check my blood sugar multiple times every hour that I worked out with her. These were the days before continuous glucose monitors. The only way to know if my blood sugar was going up, down, or remaining stable was to prick my finger and wait for the reading on the meter. There were sessions with Sue where I checked my blood sugar every ten minutes. These were the early days of learning to listen to my body. I didn't know what my body was trying to tell me, thus empirical data helped me learn. Those early sessions with Sue were slow going. I was still struggling to accept that I could become athletic while having a chronic health condition.

Slowly, over time, I began to recognize the difference between low blood sugar and regular muscle strain and athletic effort. I learned to slow down. Before checking my blood sugar, I would ask myself what I thought was happening in my body. I would set down the 10-pound weights I was lifting, and I would pause, close my eyes and listen to my body. Sue would quietly wait. Then I would prick my finger and see if my listening was on target. I wasn't right every single time, but I did learn to recognize the difference between low blood sugar and muscle effort. In fact, these days, I enjoy the effort of lifting heavy weights. Back when I started lifting with Sue, I never thought I would one day look forward to my twice weekly visits to the gym to lift weights and challenge my body to get stronger.

Doing lots of up and down movements made me dizzy and lightheaded, which felt like low blood sugar, but, as I came to find out, it wasn't. I have low blood pressure. I learned I could push myself harder than I thought. Before long, I had arm and leg muscles I never knew existed. I liked listening to the messages and wisdom my body had for me. I really liked the new strength and confidence. As my body slowly and surely got stronger, I realized I could trust it to hang in there with me. I discovered I was kinesthetically strong, not just mentally strong.

Once I had started working out with Sue on a regular and consistent basis, I was in the Stages of Change called Maintenance. This is the stage where we are keeping up the change that has been made. Please note, given a new life challenge, it is very likely and very possible that you, as I have, will move around in the Stages of Change. Like with the Stages of Grief, give yourself grace. Use these two tools, The Stages of Grief and The Stages of Change, as information to help you know yourself as you gather your courage to become an endurance athlete.

DECISION TIME

It turns out that when you get a diagnosis of a chronic health condition, you get to make a few decisions. Maybe not immediately, since a diagnosis initially throws your life into chaos.

It's important to let yourself go through the various stages of grief. Your life has changed. Your identity as a person is different than it was. Before making big decisions, allow yourself a moment to process and take it in.

I spent a few years adjusting to my diabetes diagnosis. In fact, it wasn't until I went to diabetes camp, and met other people my age who had type 1 diabetes, that I finally felt like diabetes wasn't an immediate death sentence. The relative ease I expected my life to have was gone. It wasn't until I met others who were navigating the challenges of type 1 with relative optimism that I realized I could make a decision about how I handled it.

CANCER, CHOICES TO MAKE

I have had a few opportunities to navigate a difficult health diagnosis. When I was thirty-nine and had just ridden my bike 400 miles up and down the mountains of Colorado, I found out I had breast cancer, for the first time. That diagnosis also forced me to make a decision about how I would proceed with life. The shock of the diagnosis was stunning. Breast cancer doesn't run in my family, and up until that point, no one on my mother's or father's side of the family had ever had breast cancer. Type 1 diabetes made sense, given my family history. Breast cancer felt like an arrow hit me from out of the dark.

The cancer world moves with the speed of lightning. Navigators help get multiple appointments scheduled in record time. Every part of my body was prodded and scanned. Thankfully I had a strong acupuncture system set up and I had excellent health insurance, because all those scans and prods are not cheap.

CANCER TREATMENTS

I made the decision to approach my cancer treatments the way I had approached training for that 400-mile bike ride across Colorado. The treatments coming up were a lumpectomy to remove the tumor in my breast, followed by chemotherapy, followed by radiation therapy. I had trained for the bike ride for nearly a year, participated in the event, and succeeded at finishing with a smile on my face and a strong sense of accomplishment.

I knew the value of always having someone go to the doctor with me to take notes and be another set of ears. I found a new notebook, and I kept all the cancer information in a specific canvas bag so that everything would be easily accessible for all who were going to help me. In preparation for the start of chemotherapy, I consulted with my endocrinologist about what might happen with my blood sugars with the drugs they were going to give me. Many of the drugs they gave me were to keep me from getting excessively nauseous from the chemo drugs, so I could still function. I knew I would need lots of help for the day of the chemo infusion and the one–three days after each infusion. I was on a two-week cycle for the chemo, meaning it was fast and furious. To keep my red blood cell count up, I had to give myself an injection midway through the two weeks. Due to having type 1 diabetes, and being very comfortable with giving myself injections, they let me do these red blood cell booster shots myself. The one bummer about this injection was that the drug going into my abdomen hurt like burning fire. I did lots of deep breathing while giving myself those shots.

NETWORK OF SUPPORT

I had a wide network of people willing to help me manage my chemo treatments. I made arrangements with eight sets of friends to come help for each of the scheduled eight chemo sessions. Most sets of friends came for a four-day visit. They arrived a day before chemo to acclimate to what was going to happen the next day. Then they were with me, driving me to and from the infusion site, and they hung out and socialized for the four-hour chemo infusion session.

That first chemo session threw me over and under the bus, meaning I really didn't know what to expect. They weighed me right when I arrived at the session. That's because the amount of chemo drugs they give to each person is directly related to your body mass. Essentially, they want to give you enough drugs to kill the random cancer cells drifting around in the body, but not so much that the drugs kill you. The infusion went fairly smoothly. I had a port installed in my upper arm and that worked well. None of the chemo drugs got on my skin, which apparently could have singed my skin. They gave me a number of steroids to help my body process the chemo drugs. They dramatically raised my blood sugar. I had to more than double my background insulin, which helped keep my blood sugars from going completely off the chart.

My friend Ara came to Denver to help me navigate chemo round one. Having her there was a godsend, since about three or four hours after I got home the nausea hit me hard. I had not eaten anything since lunch that day, which was before I had the chemo infusion. What little I had in my body came out with a vengeance. I had dry heaves for over twelve hours. I spent the majority of the night on the bathroom floor. I slept very little. What snatches of sleep I did get was on a towel on the floor. Every once in a while, I attempted to drink some water and soon after I drank, I threw it up. They had given me anti-nausea suppositories. After about six hours of continuous throwing up, I finally used one. That too was a new experience. But none of the pills they gave me to swallow would stay in my body. The next morning, we called the oncology office to discuss my situation and they correctly suspected that I was dramatically dehydrated, and they insisted I come in and get a saline transfusion. The drugs and the throwing up had begun to make me extremely disoriented. It was a good thing Ara was there to drive me to the hospital for that needed transfusion. They gave me a few additional anti-nausea drugs to help me navigate it all. Additionally, they took a lot of notes about my response, so they could make adjustments for chemo round two.

Ara took lots of notes in my cancer notebook about managing my insulin and blood sugars during the days after chemo. I ate virtually nothing for three days but still needed twice the insulin due to the steroids. My ability to have coherent conversations was quite limited due to the struggle my body and mind were navigating as they processed the drugs. Thankfully, Ara was there to support and help me. On about day four my mind resurfaced. My appetite didn't fully return, but I realized I was once again wanting to eat, and I could keep the food in my body.

SHORT EXERCISE BOUTS

At this point, I took short walks. I set up my bicycle on the trainer in the living room, and I rode for thirty to forty minutes. I didn't pedal fast, but what mattered to me was that I moved my body. I hung posters of Lance Armstrong and the US Postal Cycling Team that raced at the Tour de France. Remember, this was in 2004, well before we understood and knew that Lance and his cycling team were using drugs to be successful. In my mind he was a cancer-surviving athlete that served as a role model for me as I endured.

I also hung a poster of my cycling coach Nicole Freedman and her team of pro women cyclists. As I pedaled slowly on my bike in the living room, I visualized myself as a successful endurance athlete. The frame I put on this chemo experience was that this was a sixteen-week endurance event that I would accomplish. I visualized the chemo finding every and all random cancer cells and trapping them and zapping them.

Chemo round two went much more smoothly than round one. They gave me more and stronger anti-nausea drugs, and that made a positive difference. I didn't throw up. I was super disoriented and discombobulated, and I couldn't carry on a coherent conversation for two days. Again, I also didn't eat for three days. I again needed a bit more than double the insulin. Thankfully I could sleep, which I did nearly round the clock for three days. My sense of smell was activated to a new level, and the smell of cooking food caused profound waves of nausea to roll through my body. Thankfully, the friends there to help me were okay eating take-out food on my front porch swing while I hung out in my bedroom with a fan on so I couldn't smell the food.

DECISIONS AND COMMITMENTS

Throughout my cancer treatment, I made choices that greatly impacted my life: how I chose to view it in my own mind as an endurance challenge, how I organized myself, how I surrounded myself with a reliable support network, and how I chose to continue my other goals as much as possible by exercising when I could. This approach to cancer helped solidify my identity as an athlete who was faced with cancer. Making a decision and then a commitment about how I would approach this difficult health challenge gave me my power back and it opened up space within myself to feel hope.

The decision about how you will handle your disease is a decision you can revisit often. Allow yourself time to go through the Stages of Grief. If you have enough awareness, step outside of yourself and see if you can name the stage of grief you are in. I find that if I slow down, breathe quietly, and look inside, I notice where I am. That gives me a sense of control of what's happening in a seemingly uncontrollable situation. Often that attention helps me move through that stage with more ease. While you are in a powerful stage of grief, it is nearly impossible to set big athletic goals. Feeling the emotions and allowing the grief can be enough.

Then, as you allow and breathe, things will again shift. You can then consciously notice the Stage of Change you are in. I remind you of this because, again, knowing yourself and where you are will empower you from the inside out. When you know where you are in the Stages of Change, you can coach yourself to make athletic goals. I believe in you. So much. It's why I wrote this book for you.

TRY THIS

Journal

Step 1: Take a moment and write down your challenge. Do you have a chronic disease? Do you have a weight challenge? Do you think you're too old? Whatever it is, write it down. Write all of it down. Putting it on paper helps create a bit of space around it.

Step 2: Think about the Stages of Grief: denial, anger, bargaining, depression, acceptance. Consider if you are in one or two or three of these stages of grief around your challenge. If you are, take a moment and describe how that is showing up for you. Do you have enough support? Would you like more support? Can you give yourself some space and some grace for wherever you are? If you're in a difficult stage of grief, stop here and be kind to yourself. This might be enough for today.

Step 3: Take a moment and review the Stages of Change model. The Stages are: Pre-Contemplation, Contemplation, Preparation, Action, and Maintenance. What stage do you think you are at regarding becoming an athlete? Why? Capture these musings in your journal. Take a moment and think about how you might gather more information and coach yourself into the stage of action.

Action

Step 4: Do a short meditation and ask inside yourself, "Inner Healer, are you there?" Notice what you observe. If you are meeting your Inner Healer for the first time, thank them for guiding you to find this book.

Notes

1. June, "Understanding the Seven Stages of Grief and Chronic Illness," NAFC Fitness Certification, October 21, 2021, https://nafconline.com/nafc-blog/understanding-the-seven-stages-of-grief-and-chronic-illness. See also Paula, "Processing a New Diagnosis of Chronic Illness? The Stages of Grief," Dochas Psychological Services, Inc., 2022, https://www.dochaspsych.com/blog-processing-a-new-diagnosis-of-chronic-illness-the-stages-of-grief.

2. "What Is the 'Inner Healing Intelligence'?" Entheo Medicine, https://entheomedicine.org/2021/04/what-is-the-inner-healing-intelligence. Another resource is Lissa Rankin, MD. She teaches how to find your Inner Pilot Light, which is another name for your Inner Healer. Her websites are https://lissarankin.com and http://innerpilotlight.com.

3. "The Transtheoretical Model: An Integrative Model of Behavior Change," ProChange Behavior Solutions, https://prochange.com/transtheoretical-model-of-behavior-change.

4. Ibid.

Resources

Radical Acceptance, by Tara Brach, www.tarabrach.com

Patient defiance or how to engage patients in health decision-making: Rebecca E Say and Richard Thomson, "The importance of patient preferences in treatment decisions—challenges for doctors," BMJ (Clinical research ed.), 327(7414), 542–545. https://doi.org/10.1136/bmj.327.7414.542, https://www.ncbi.nlm.nih.gov/pmc/articles/PMC192849.

CHAPTER 3

FEAR & OBSTACLES

WHAT GETS IN YOUR WAY

"Obstacles don't have to stop you.
If you run into a wall, don't turn around
and give up. Figure out how to climb it,
go through it, or work around it."

—*MICHAEL JORDAN*

DO YOU EVER RUN UP AGAINST THE FEELING OR THOUGHT that you can't be an athlete? That things in your life—your age, your weight, your health, your trauma—are just too challenging to overcome? It's easy to get derailed and want to give up before even sorting out what's real and true for you. Becoming an endurance athlete begins with the decision to become one. The deciding process, when done with honesty and intent, cements your commitment and sets you up for success.

After you make the mental decision to become an athlete, the next step is to define your obstacle, or if you're like me, your obstacles. Yes, I've got more than one obstacle. As I was starting out, if it wasn't one thing holding me back, it was another. Paint a clear picture of what challenges or problems you believe you're up against, what you need to solve. Then you can define what assistance you need. Often our problems become so daunting in our minds that they take on lives of their own, consuming us to the point of overwhelm. Quickly paralysis sets in. Our pursuit is over before it's even begun. This chapter will cover defining our obstacles, confronting our fears, and then reframing those fears.

NOTICE THE FEAR

I live in St. Paul, Minnesota, and a few years ago in an effort to make peace with the endless wintertime snow and cold, I went to a local upcycle gear store and purchased a pair of used, good condition, classic cross-country skis, boots, and poles. I figured having the gear was a good first step. The challenge was that I couldn't remember how to cross-country ski, and the fear swallowed me up every time I considered going out and giving it a try. I was afraid I would fall and hurt myself. I was afraid of looking stupid. I had no idea where I should and could go to ski safely. My fear shut me down before I could get out the door. Additionally, at the time I purchased those skis, I did not have any friends who liked to cross-country ski. Essentially, I was stuck in my fear.

A few Decembers later, after the skis sat in the corner gathering dust, my triathlon friend Monica emailed a few of us and told us she was taking cross-country ski lessons at Mount Como in Saint Paul, Minnesota. Did any of us want to join her? I jumped at the chance. Three of us joined. Delightfully, we three were the majority in the small class, and the instructors were patient, good-humored college students with lots of energy and willingness to explain how to ski over and over again. In a few weeks, I was pleased to discover I had fallen in love again with cross-country skiing. Gliding over the snow evoked in me an all-over peacefulness. The glide feels like a quiet connectedness to all of nature.

Take a moment and think about the sport you want to undertake. What fears do you notice? Where in your body do you notice the fear living? What happens when you notice the fear? Do you, like me, get stuck, lost, overwhelmed? For now, just notice the fear, and give it a bit of kindness and non-judgmental space.

DEFINE THE OBSTACLE

My friend and cycling coach, Nicole Freedman, started bike racing while attending Stanford University. Nicole quickly discovered that she was an excellent cyclist and had the potential to win races. As part of her training, Nicole's coach had her get a VO2 max test, or maximal oxygen consumption test, to measure how much oxygen she used during intense exercise. This test is considered one of the best indicators of cardiovascular fitness and aerobic endurance and it is thought that it can predict your athletic potential. Nicole was surprised and disappointed to find out that her VO2 max was considered suboptimal for an endurance athlete.

Nicole loved cycling and, not to be deterred, wanted to create for herself a life of bike racing. To her way of thinking, if her genetic predisposition for VO2 max wasn't high, she would learn what she could do (what actions she could take) to increase her fitness. She became an expert in sport periodization training and sports nutrition. She read everything she could get her hands on about both concepts. Her goal was to understand and implement both so she could enhance her performance.

Her persistence and knowledge paid off. Nicole won the USA National Women's Road Race Championship one year and the USA National Women's Criterion Championship the next. These two types of races require different athletic skills; thus, Nicole's accomplishment is especially impressive. A road race involves riding long distances day after day, with a team of riders. Road racing covers a range of distances from 30 miles to over 100 miles in a given day, over roads where few spectators are watching and cheering. As a result, road racing requires intense mental focus, dependence on your teammates, and your own ability to navigate physical pain and challenges.

A criterion race is a specified number of laps on a course that's often made up of several city blocks that are closed to traffic, making them easy and fun for spectators to watch. Criterions, often called crits, are done at very high speeds and with the cyclists riding very close to one another. Since they are done on city streets, the racing involves lots of cornering, which can cause crashes to happen very quickly. Nicole went on to qualify for the 2000 USA Olympic women's cycling team that competed in Sydney, Australia. For more than twelve years, Nicole raced on and managed a professional women's cycling team, winning dozens of races. She found a successful work-around to her VO2 max levels. She defined her obstacle. Then she found strategies to overcome the obstacle. You too can do this.

After noticing your own fear, think about the obstacles you face. As you shift your thinking from your fears to your obstacles, you might notice more space within yourself to begin to imagine solutions. I find that fears are emotions, and obstacles are problems that can be solved. In the case of my early cross-country ski experience, I had fears that resulted in obstacles. In Nicole's case, she had fear about her fitness level, which led her to redefine it as a challenge to overcome. In both cases, we found solutions.

Often, before you can get to solutions, you will need to do one more step.

CONFRONTING FEAR

On New Year's Eve a few years ago, I set the resolution to notice and directly confront my fears as they arose. This resolution came in handy when, that year, I broke my ankle a week after my birthday, the first time in my life I'd ever broken a bone. The break happened two weeks before I was to ride my bicycle 100 miles on the twenty-fifth anniversary of the American Diabetes Association Tour de Cure. I had trained sixteen weeks for this ride and felt strong and ready. Doing the ride was how I wanted to commemorate living successfully with diabetes for thirty-five years.

Within a week of the break, fear set in with a vengeance. Initially, I wasn't sure what the fear was; I just noticed I was holding my breath often. I also observed that it was extremely difficult to accept and ask for assistance from the friends who offered help. In the spirit of confronting my fears, I sat down and took a series of deep breaths. I calmed my body down. I closed my eyes. I asked my guardian angels to guide and support me. Then I turned and asked my fears to please step into the light. I told them that I wanted to understand them.

Fears, not surprisingly, aren't fond of the light. They much prefer skirting around the subconscious and messing with us in the background. So, I waited. And waited. While I waited,

I kept breathing calmly. Finally, one big fear stepped into the arena of my mind and said, "No one will ever want to be with you. Now you can't walk. You can't even walk your dog. You can't push a grocery cart. Why would anyone ever love you? You might never again be able to exercise. Why don't you just give up? Besides, now that you can't exercise at all, you're going to get super fat."

I had to keep breathing and stay calm in the face of this fear's viciousness. I felt my belly clench and my heart started to pound. Deep breathing and asking my guardian angels to help me allowed me to calm the tension and anxiety that crept up. I let the fear dance around a bit more and wear itself out. When it was done ranting, I asked, "Is there any more?" It let me know that it was done, for now.

I then told it I was grateful it let me know how worried and worthless it felt. I told the fear that it was safe now, that I was glad it found the courage to tell me its truth. I reassured the fear that I was listening closely to it and that I would make every effort to listen as we moved forward.

That shocked the fear. I noticed it shrinking. Slowly, it stopped looking prickly and sharp. I kept breathing deeply. I realized, as I felt and contemplated what it had told me, that much of my strength post-healing from the sexual abuse I survived as a child was through my identity as an athlete. Losing contact with that identity in the face of my broken ankle awakened dormant fears, and those fears came out with a shaming bite.

HOW FEAR HOLDS US BACK

Every single human being experiences fear at some point: fear of the unknown, fear of others, fear of ourselves, fear of what's behind a closed door. I helped start the Link Crew program, a high school orientation program run by the Boomerang Project. In Link Crew, we tell a story about a prisoner and fear. This prisoner knows he is going to be executed. He is brought out to the prison yard where the execution will be held. The prisoner sees five guards who all have guns standing in a line. The captain of the guards steps toward the prisoner and asks, "You have a choice. You can take either the blindfold or this key, which would you like?" The prisoner ponders a moment, and asks, "What does the key unlock?" The guard holds up the key and points to a locked door on the side of the prison wall and says, "It's for that door."

The prisoner ponders long and hard, and then reaches for the blindfold and puts it on. A moment later, five shots ring out and the prisoner drops to the ground. As the guards are leaving, one of them asks the captain, "You always offer the key and the blindfold. They always take the blindfold. What does that door open up to?" The captain shakes his head and says, "That door leads to freedom. The prisoners take the known over the unknown."

This story resonates with me on so many levels. Doing what is known, even if the known will kill us, is often easier than taking a chance on the unknown. So many of us are prisoners of the known. We won't risk doing what is unknown. I often have to remind myself of this story to help me gather my courage to do the unknown. You are worth taking a moment to examine your fear, define your obstacles, and finally, confront your fear. Staying with your fear might mean you'll miss out on life-transforming adventures.

MY FIRST TRIATHLON

When I did my first triathlon, after finishing chemotherapy and radiation therapy for my first round of breast cancer, I had to recite over and over, "I can do this. I am an athlete." I hadn't trained for that first triathlon, so during it, I was going on pure willpower and guts. Not something I recommend.

Cancer shredded my confidence and worked hard to destroy the progress I had gained doing the Bicycle Tour of Colorado the summer before I was diagnosed with cancer. Finishing that first triathlon was a huge celebration of survival. Chemo and radiation trounced me to the ground and even so, I made it through, much to my relief. At that first triathlon, people cheered me for being a cancer survivor and for being out there racing. The feeling of appreciation and acknowledgement for what I had survived and accomplished soothed its way into the Swiss cheese holes in my sense of self. I felt a part of a community that celebrated athletic accomplishment. This was a community I wanted to belong to going forward. To my toes I felt like I had finally found my people.

THE SHADOW REARS ITS HEAD

Do you have a shadow? I'm not talking about your body shape that appears on the concrete when the sun is shining, but what Swiss psychiatrist Carl Jung called the "unknown dark side of the personality."[1] The unknown dark side of the personality is the part of us that holds our fear. Getting inspired and motivated to exercise can cause our shadow side and our fears to rear up. I know for me that the hiding and festering of my fear can become very uncomfortable, causing inaction and internal cowering.

The shadow contains all the parts of ourselves that we try to hide or deny, the dark aspects we believe are unacceptable to family, friends, and, most important, ourselves. Stuffed deeply within our subconscious, hidden from others and ourselves, our dark side sends simple, damaging messages: "There is something wrong with me." "I am not OK." "I am unlovable." "I am undeserving." "I am not worthy." "I am bad."

I have struggled for much of my life with the deep, dark shadow that I am not lovable and worthy: I am not enough. For much of my early adulthood, I didn't understand this shadow side of myself, and I didn't understand the fears that would come out at surprising moments. It would come out when I joined friends at a picnic, and someone would suggest we play kickball or frisbee. My belief that I was clumsy, ungraceful, and couldn't catch a ball or frisbee came out and shut me down. This part of me often said no to even attending gatherings for fear I'd be asked to play. I didn't even have the confidence to sit out when asked to join in. I figured not even going to the gathering was a better option. I shut myself out of being with good people.

Thankfully, I found my way to profound therapeutic processes and wise guides. I found Holotropic Breathwork®2, hypnotherapy, and somatic healing (which is healing that takes into account the nervous system). In Holotropic Breathwork, I learned to allow my shadow side to speak to me. I learned how to clear internal space within myself to witness my past traumas without judging myself. Rather than shrink from my shadow, I learned to understand it rather than project it onto the people and world around me.

DESIRE TO GET BACK IN MY BODY

I didn't understand my shadow self because I did not consciously remember that I was a sexual abuse survivor. After I graduated from college in Saint Paul, Minnesota, I moved to Santa Cruz, California, to become a high school Spanish teacher. While there, I experienced the 1989 Loma Prieta earthquake. The trauma of the earthquake kicked up memories of earlier trauma from my life. My memory cracked open, and I remembered being sexually abused as a child. The memories dramatically interrupted my daily life. I thought I was going crazy. It was as if I had a movie playing inside my head at all hours of the day and night, a movie I didn't want to see.

Prior to the earthquake, I had had no recollection of such trauma. Suddenly, the images were vividly clear and the feelings in my body shouted loudly, confirming the memories. My Inner Healer kept assuring me it was unlikely I was making it up. I was overwhelmed. I found myself shaking at odd times of the day and night, and my sleeping was radically disrupted. I knew I needed help to navigate this new territory. I opened myself to finding assistance, which is a critical first step in healing and transformation.

I found childhood sexual abuse expert Ellen Bass, author of one of the first books about sexual abuse, *The Courage to Heal*.[3] As my good fortune would have it, Ellen lived in Santa Cruz and (along with her art therapist colleague, Amy Pine) had a weekly support group for sexual abuse survivors. Upon joining the group, my sexual abuse healing journey began.

Over time, I came to understand that the perpetrators were my father, my grandfather, and a babysitter I went to when I was four years old. The abuse started when I was nine months old and ended when I was eleven. Long periods of time went by when nothing happened. During these "nothing happening" times, I was in an extreme fight-or-flight readiness phase. Being on high alert made me become hyperaware of every environment I was in, which continues to serve me in my professional work. It serves me that without much effort, I can tune into what is happening in a new environment. Unfortunately, it also caused my nervous system to work too hard.

Part of my fear of exercising, I came to realize, was the result of staying out of touch with my body most of my life. As a child, I'd had to dissociate, or disengage, from my physical being to endure abuse that I was too young to understand and too powerless to stop. I'd shut down physical sensation at a deep level. As an adult, exercise put me firmly back in my body, somewhere I was afraid to be. What had been an essential survival tool when I was a child had become a barrier now that I was an adult who needed and wanted to start exercising.

Fears I had carried inside since I was a child became less frightening as I wrote them down, which I did as part of the therapeutic journaling process I did with Ellen, Amy, and the one-on-one therapists I saw for extra support. The memories of the early experiences slowly lost their power. As I wrote, I cried. I cried for all that I had lost by being detached from my body most of my life. For the first time, I let the tears fall. Tears, like exercise, put me in my body. Emotions live in our body. My survival strategy had always been to exist only in my intellect. Now it was time to apply my intellect to solving my health problem, namely that I didn't have any sort of regular exercise practice or routine.

I have had to endure difficult times. You can no doubt relate, since difficult times are part of the human condition. In my case, some of the difficulties hurt my body and heart so badly that I left my body in order to endure.

ESCAPE THE PAIN

My early survival strategy was to escape feeling the pain. Thankfully, I didn't become addicted to drugs, alcohol, or food. The main way I escaped was avoiding activities that put me in my body. I wore clothes that were too big. I hated doing any sports or activities that involved wearing tight or skimpy clothing. Wearing bathing suits terrified me. I was hiding. I didn't like my body, and I didn't want anyone to notice my body. There were times it seemed that my avoidance was working, but, as wise people have taught through history, the only way out is through.

Metaphorically, the idea is to take a deep breath and dive into the pain, even the past pain, feeling each strand of it. Meaning my task was to go back and explore the memories and allow my body to feel the pain. As mentioned, early on I found my way to skilled therapists. With their insights and ability to hold space for me, I found the courage to dive in and find the critical threads of healing that led me back to my heart and body. Holding space happens when someone has done enough of their own inner work to be able to be fully present for others. Chances are good you've felt the benefit of someone holding space for you. In my case, this method resulted in moving into freedom and significantly less pain.

Embracing the Shadow Isn't Easy

When it comes to exercise, you may find your shadow side rises up and tries to dissuade you from taking action. This has happened to me. In fact, it happens every year in mid-December. I get extra sleepy and really negative about my athletic plans. I overeat and often avoid my athletic friends. For a while I thought it was seasonal depression. When I identified it as my shadow, I took back my power. Now, when these symptoms show up, instead of letting the shadow take over, I sit down and have a conversation with the shadow. I welcome the shadow, and I ask it, every year, what it wants from me. Every time we have this conversation, and I attentively listen, the shadow backs down and I recover the energy for my next athletic goal.

Survivors Make Excellent Endurance Athletes

Those of us who have suffered profoundly in life are the ideal people to tackle endurance athletics. Both require tuning in to your innermost strengths. Both ask us to endure tremendous suffering and turn that suffering into something worthwhile. Time and time again, when I am out racing or participating in a long endurance event, I draw on how I have survived as a source of powerful strength. I go inward and remind myself how much I have endured. The simple act of breathing into the suffering during an athletic event allows me to create more space in my being for the suffering. Instead of working to shut down the suffering, I embrace it, allow it, welcome it, feel it all the way. I hear it within my body. I can then analyze it, determining if it's warning me in some way. If not, the allowing opens up more space, and often, more energy to carry on. You too can tap into your inner strength and ability to endure and thrive.

There are days my shadow rears its head with a ferociousness that stuns me. A few years ago, I believed a longtime friend would not notice if I didn't attend her anniversary party. It was heading into winter and my energy was low. I did not have someone to go to the party with me, and I wouldn't know many people in attendance. I had a lot of excuses. I believed she wouldn't really care or notice if I was there or not. Turns out, she did notice, and she was disappointed. When she told me, I was shocked; I didn't believe I mattered. That was my shadow.

One of the tools I've learned to help me know my shadow is operating is to pay attention when an action of a friend surprises me or jolts me. I've learned to analyze surprises and shock. Often when I reflect, I discover that my shadow has snuck in and has started to distort my reality. I've kept up with nearly weekly therapy. It is reassuring and valuable to have someone whom I can count on to help sort out the confusion and trauma from my early life and how it rears its head in my adult daily life. I am committed to continued personal growth and healing, just as I am committed to remaining fit and healthy my whole life. I need other people to help and encourage me. You too deserve to have support and guidance. If you don't yet have a therapist, I encourage you to look at the services your health insurance provides for mental health support.

The Shadow/Fear Loop

It's easy to get caught in the negative cycle of describing and feeling whatever difficulty you have. With my diabetes, I spent years telling stories of how hopeless it was for me to avoid low blood sugars when exercising. I described and overdescribed how awful it had been to witness my father have low blood sugars and almost die time and again. I relived the fear over and over. Without defining it as such, I was committed to being out of my body, so I avoided any activity that got me into my body. There were a number of times that I ended friendships with people who wanted to push me to get active. For many years I avoided relationships, because of my sexual abuse memories. I told myself how unattractive and worthless I was. Because of this, I stayed away from friendships with people that encouraged me to try dating. Fear is an easy trap to fall into. The fear loop is surprisingly comfortable, and what we find comfortable is difficult to leave.

Fear comes up at unexpected moments. Learning to be with fear and move through it is a lifelong process that takes the skill of reframing. It's a skill that I am grateful I've learned and keep practicing how to use. You too can learn how to reframe.

REFRAMING FEAR AND OBSTACLES

Early in my healing journey, I learned about reframing. The technique is easy to perform and is extremely powerful. So powerful, in fact, that sometimes, it is the only technique you need to change a belief and then a behavior. Reframing, as described by Dave Evans and Bill Burnett (two Stanford University Design School professors), is "pivoting your perspective to address a perceived problem."[4] Let's explore how you practice reframing.

When Is Reframing Useful?

Blogger Michael Davidson describes reframing as a piece of "software" to install in your mind.[5] You might not reframe everything, but you should at least be able to do it whenever a situation arises that you want to transform. It takes a moment and a bit of studying to learn how to do reframing. In my life, the skill of reframing is what helps me survive and continue to find meaning and value in challenges that otherwise might have caused me to give up and sink into depression and further suicide attempts.

Principles of Reframing and How to Do It

It's critical to know and accept these principles for reframing before trying to add reframing to your personal development toolkit. A reframe is more effective when you understand what's going on behind the skill of doing it.

The first basic principle is that events or situations do not have inherent meaning; you assign them meaning based on how you interpret the event. This can be difficult to accept, but you must. Even when something seemingly horrible happens to you, *it is only horrible because of the way you look at it.* For example, when I got my diagnosis of type 1 diabetes at age sixteen, my first reaction was, "Oh shoot, now I'm like Dad." I was sad for a few days. I still remember those tear-filled days. I lay on my bed not moving, feeling my heart break inside my chest. Then I realized I did *not* want to be like my dad, and to not be like my dad, I needed to have a different approach to my diabetes than he had. He kept his diabetes quiet, and he subjected our family to quite a bit of trauma because of his apparent desire to pretend that he didn't really have diabetes and that he didn't really need to pay close attention to what he ate and how it affected him. Instead, I wanted to view having diabetes as an opportunity to take care of myself and learn everything I could about managing it well. I reframed my diagnosis of diabetes.

This is not to make light of tragedy. It's perfectly OK to be sad when something seemingly bad occurs. That being said, even a "bad" event can be given a "good" meaning.

Every thought has a hidden "frame" behind it. The frame is your beliefs about the situation, your assumptions that are implied by your thoughts. For example, when you think, "I'll never get that promotion because I'm not an ass-kisser at work," part of the frame is the belief that only suck-ups get promoted.

Positive Intention behind Every Negative Thought

The next part of reframing is that there is a positive intention behind every negative thought. Your inner voice only expresses negativity because it wants to help you in some way. That doesn't make the thoughts right or acceptable, of course, but it does mean your inner voice isn't an enemy to be resisted. This one can be a bit tricky to understand. When I reframed my diabetes diagnosis, it was in part in rebellion to how my dad had handled his diabetes. Upon reflection, I could have left it at that: I was rebelling.

Instead, I continued to examine my motivation. As I've mentioned, I made friends early in my life with my inner wisdom, what I call my Inner Healer. That inner voice initially used rebellion with me, because as a teenager, I understood rebellion. Rebellion caused action, which was the goal the Inner Healer wanted me to achieve. Later, as I continued my healing journey, I realized my Inner Healer always has my good intentions and well-being in mind. I might not always immediately understand what my Inner Healer's intention is, but I can take a few minutes to reflect and consider, without judgment, what might be behind the intention. If I do this, I have found that, every single time, I can trust and rely on my Inner Healer to have my back. Discovering that there is wisdom and caring in the universe for me allows deep healing. That has made the skill of reframing that much more valuable.

By finding the positive intentions behind your thoughts, you can work *with* your mind to find a positive reframe. Notably, I found a way to act, which is what my Inner Healer wanted by inviting me to rebel. That's far more effective than chastising yourself for having negative thoughts in the first place. At its simplest, reframing involves just two steps: observing a negative thought and then replacing it with a positive one.

OBSERVING YOUR NEGATIVE THOUGHTS

Negative thoughts pop up in our minds about a gazillion times a day. They often follow the same few patterns and usually sneak by unquestioned. It's time to put a stop to this. To help you observe your negative thoughts, keep a thought journal, or use the rubber band technique, or both.

Keep a Thought Journal

Always keep a small notepad in your pocket or bag so it's available at all times. I find taking notes on my phone to be too slow, but you're free to try it. Anytime you have a negative thought, write it down. This stops your negative thought in its tracks, allowing you to analyze it and, over time, notice your most common problem areas or limiting beliefs. One of the negative thoughts I've been tracking in my thought journal is how often I tell myself I will never have enough money. My thought journal (I use a tiny notepad) is filled with the date, time, and circumstances when I have the thought that I will never have enough money. Slowly, I'm coming to observe that the context around when I have that thought is important to pay attention to. Meaning that often I have negative money thoughts when I'm around people who have access to much more money than I do. I notice I start to focus on how lacking I am in comparison. That starts a negative spiral. Slowly, I'm teaching myself to not compare and instead to focus on how much I do have.

Rubber Band Technique

This method feels a little silly at first, but it's one of the fastest ways to change a behavior. Wear a rubber band around your wrist. I wear a black hair tie, because it blends with the bracelets I wear on my wrist, so people don't notice it. It should be tight enough to stay on and make a nice snap when pulled but loose enough that it's comfortable and won't break. Any time you have a negative thought, give the rubber band a snap. Like writing it down, this stops a negative thought in its tracks immediately, but also conditions you to have fewer negative thoughts in the future.

Recognizing your negative thoughts is key to being able to successfully reframe them.

Replacing Negative Thoughts with Positive Ones

Knowing how to replace negative thoughts with positive thoughts takes a bit of practice. At times, I've stood in front of a mirror and said negative thoughts out loud to myself and then shook my body and practiced replacing the negative thought using the methods listed below. It can be fun to practice changing your thoughts. Really.

Use milder wording. This one is easy, and you can start doing it immediately. Words matter, and if your thought is worded more mildly, you won't feel as badly. For example, if you were to think, *I really hate that guy*, you would feel worse than if you thought, *I'm not a fan of that guy*. Go with the second one. When I catch myself having a negative thought about my finances, I have a few reframes I immediately use, such as, "I don't have a lot of money in my bank account today, and that can and will change very soon." I also tell myself, "Remember, you've always had enough money to feed and house yourself and to go on fun vacations. Trust the universe and your talent and skill; financial wellness and abundance is happening."

"What is the best way for me to accomplish this?" When facing a challenge or fear, asking yourself this question helps you focus on the solution rather than the problem. "Best way" implies that there are multiple ways around the problem and focuses on the positive. When the thought that I will never have enough money comes up, I now ask myself, "What is the best way for me to bring in more income?" I've discovered a few lucrative side hustles as a result of choosing a brainstorming, problem-solving mindset.

"What can I learn from this?" Instead of having a problem, you now have a way to improve yourself. Every challenge is also an opportunity to learn, so take advantage of it. When I'm managing my finances and I notice I'm going to run out of money before my next paycheck, instead of beating myself up, I've learned to ask myself, "What can I learn from this?" Amazingly, this approach has helped me be more careful with my spending before I run out of money, instead of shutting myself down in despair for not having enough.

Challenge your assumptions. Try to figure out the frame behind your thought. Chances are, you have a limiting belief that's encouraging you to think negatively about your situation. This limiting belief is based on assumptions you've made that probably aren't true. When you find reasons why they aren't true, you chip away at the beliefs causing the negative thoughts. This is the most powerful long-term reframing technique, and it is far more effective if you've been keeping a thought journal. I come from a family that taught me to believe in scarcity. That limiting belief is the frame behind most of my thinking that "I have no money" and "I will never have enough income." In my case, this limiting belief is not even true! I have rarely directly experienced profound scarcity. It was worth the time and energy to challenge this hidden assumption.

What is my value to the world? When faced with a negative thought or belief, take a step back and look at the bigger picture. In the moment I confronted my fears after breaking my ankle, I quietly sat there breathing, and ideas for possible actions regarding my broken ankle started to come to me. First, I thought about what value I offer the world besides being an endurance athlete. Value that means something to me. Value that I value. What came to mind: Trustworthy. Consistent. Reliable. Energetic. Having integrity. Loving. Organized. Efficient. Enthusiastic. After listing these values, I asked the fear, "Do you hear the value I bring to the world? I offer the world more than my endurance and athleticism." I could feel the fear resisting, but it was listening. When I stood up, something had shifted in my left leg, the side on which I'd broken my ankle. It felt stronger, like the fear had been living in my leg and had loosened its grip.

Fitness Waxes and Wanes, Move with the Fear That Arises

Finding my way back to wellness after breaking my ankle reminded me that athleticism, like many things in life, is a spiral, not a straight line. Fitness and wellness in general work this way too. Identifying my obstacles and confronting my fears will likely be something I will have to do again and again, as new obstacles and new fears arise. I like things to move forward in straight lines; I like learning a lesson and being done with it. Unfortunately, that's not how things work in life and health, darn it.

In fact, I've now broken my ankle twice. The second time I broke it, I slipped on an icy sidewalk in early April, right after a surprise snowfall that caused much of the snow to melt and then freeze again. I decided to go out for a quick run. I didn't wear my DueNorth ice traction aids on my shoes. Bad decision. About half a mile into the run I slipped hard. Like the first time I broke the ankle, I felt a crack. I immediately knew I had broken it again. Unlike the first time, I knew I needed help as quickly as I could get it. I did not attempt to walk home, which I did the first time. Thankfully someone driving by saw me fall. She stopped her car, and asked if she could help. I called out, "Yes, please."

She pulled her SUV over and helped me hobble to her car. Then she drove me the half-mile home. I called my friend Linda, who had helped me the first time. Linda drove me to the orthopedic urgent care, as she had with the first ankle break.

As luck would have it, the same doctor was on duty. It was two years later, and he remembered me. He was surprised that the ankle broke in the same place it had previously. This second time I also broke a bone in my foot. On went the boot, and I made an appointment to see the orthopedic surgeon a few days later. Once again, no surgery and no hardware were needed. I did need to get the knee scooter again, and everything I'd learned about staying fit while not able to walk, run, or bike went into effect once again. I needed to talk to my fears again, but in this second go around, it wasn't as difficult.

IN AND OUT OF THE STAGES OF CHANGE

It's reassuring to know that I can rely on skills I've learned over the years and to reflect on where I am in the Stages of Change cycle. After breaking my ankle, both times I got flung into nearly no exercise for eight weeks and had to use the knee scooter to get around. During that phase, I realized I wasn't going to be able to ride my bike or walk much for a while. I started to brainstorm what other kinds of exercise I could do.

I was in the Contemplation stage. When I figured out that water aerobics could work but I didn't have a pool membership, I went to the YWCA and applied for a scholarship. At that point, I moved into Preparation. Getting an OK from my doctor to be in the pool and attending my water aerobics class, I entered the Action stage. As the ideas started flowing, I also realized I enjoy dancing, so I looked up chair dancing. Turns out there are all kinds of free videos on YouTube of instructors who offer a wide variety of chair dancing options, music, and happy energy. One of my favorites is Paul Eugene.[6] Look him up if you're ever injured and need a low-impact exercise option.

Knowing what Stage of Change I'm in allows me to feel in control of a situation that feels very out of control. It moves me from feeling like a victim of bad circumstances to feeling empowered and managing my destiny.

It's about defining your fears and obstacles. Confronting your fears and obstacles, and then moving into reframing them. If you find it helpful, you can use the Stages of Change tool to solidify within yourself that you are in control, and to remind yourself that you aren't a victim of the current challenge. It's breathing into your wisdom and reminding yourself that you are smart and can figure out options and paths.

TRY THIS

Journal

Part 1: Define the obstacles and fears
Take a moment to describe and define your obstacles and fears. Do this on paper, which removes the obstacle from the space in your mind where it festers and grows. Very likely, by writing it down, you will realize that the problem isn't as consuming as you thought. The obstacle can be overcome. A solution exists.

In particular, explore your fears and obstacles related to becoming an endurance athlete.

Part 2: Reframe the fears and obstacles
Rewrite your obstacles and fears at the head of this new entry. Describe the obstacles and what emotions you have around each obstacle. Imagine addressing the fear. What would you say to it? Begin to reframe. Which parts of reframing can you

do right now? What additional reframing can you do? Begin now to identify the help you need to overcome the obstacle. Make a list of people you know who might be able to help you. If there's no one to help you, think about how you could figure out solutions. Begin to describe what action steps you will take. Keep noticing all that you know how to do. Remind yourself that you are smart and capable.

Action

Give yourself time, space, and lots of grace

Paying attention to your obstacles and fears, and then working to reframe them is hard work. Be gentle with yourself. If you can, find support. You, your health, and your overall well-being is worth taking the time.

Notes

1. Carl Jung in "Shadow (psychology)," Wikipedia, https://en.wikipedia .org/wiki/Shadow_(psychology).
2. "About Holotropic Breathwork," GROF Transpersonal Training, http://www.holotropic.com/holotropic-breathwork/about-holotropic -breathwork.
3. See Ellen Bass at https://www.ellenbass.com.
4. Dave Evans and Bill Burnett, *Designing Your Life: How to Build a Well-Lived, Joyful Life* (KNOPF, 2021). See also http://lifedesignlab .stanford.edu/resources, https://designingyour.life, and http://changingminds.org/techniques/general/reframing.htm.
5. See Michael Davidson at https://michael-davidson.com.
6. See Paul Eugene at https://www.youtube.com/@PaulEugene.

Resources

Diabetes Training Camp: https://diabetestrainingcamp.com

Sports Nutrition: Phil Mafatone, https://philmaffetone.com

Big Hairy Audacious Goals: https://www.jimcollins.com/article_topics /articles/BHAG.html

Widen the Window: Training Your Brain and Body to Thrive During Stress and Recover from Trauma, by Elizabeth A. Stanley, PhD. https:// elizabeth-stanley.com/books-publications/widen-the-window

What Happened To You? Conversations on Trauma, Resilience, and Healing by Bruce D. Perry, MD, PhD; and Oprah Winfrey

CHAPTER 4

MOTIVATION

GET OUT THE DOOR

"The most common way people give up their power is by thinking they don't have any."

—ALICE WALKER

YOU UNDERSTAND YOUR OBSTACLES; NOW IT'S TIME TO understand motivation. After all, understanding your obstacles likely won't get you moving. My hope is that in understanding your obstacles and fears, you can discover your motivation and inspiration so you will get moving. In a broad sense, there are two types of motivation: intrinsic motivation and extrinsic motivation. Understanding both will go a long way in helping you get off the couch and out the door.

I have a good relationship with motivation. I think that's because early on I had to look inward to find my reason for getting going every day. The sexual abuse stopped when I was about eleven and my memory stuffed any recollection of having been abused. What lingered in my being was the sense that at any moment something awfully bad could and likely would happen to me. An edge of caution and hesitation hovered over and around me twenty-four hours a day. That took a massive amount of energy. It also made me distrustful of other people. Thankfully, I knew to look inside, even as a new teenager. School was a safe place, so I got involved. School was an external motivation for me. In eighth grade, I helped organize a trip via train out to Big Sky, Montana. A handful of students and I put together a school store, selling various junk food items (ironic, I know, given my adult passion for healthy eating), which allowed us to fundraise a significant percentage of the funds needed for the trip. We were going to downhill ski for a week in Montana. I had no idea, at all, how to downhill ski. To get out of the house and learn this new skill, two of my friends and I signed up for downhill ski lessons. Going to ski lessons for this ski trip was a combination of external and internal motivation. External because I didn't want to make a fool of myself in Montana. Internal because I quickly discovered the joy and fun of playing in the snow.

I tentatively learned how to downhill ski during lessons on a very small hill near my house. I say "tentatively" because the lessons were filled with laughter and falling over and over. When we got to the majestic Rocky Mountains of Montana, I was impressed by the sweeping beauty. I skied the easiest slopes and thoroughly enjoyed the time away from home with friends and classmates. My love of travel was ignited. Travel and service to a cause bigger than me became clear reasons to get out of bed every day.

Let's explore these two types of motivation.

INTRINSIC MOTIVATION

Intrinsic motivation comes from inside you (internal); your interest in and pleasure from doing something isn't dependent on outside factors. You find the task rewarding. Traveling to new places and being of service are examples of intrinsic motivation that work well for me. The discovery of new places brings me great joy, as does being of service to people.

Intrinsic motivation is lasting and powerful and comes in handy when no one believes in you and when you start to doubt yourself. It is dependent on the stories you tell yourself. As mentioned, I am the survivor of a challenging childhood. As a result, I realized early on that I needed support and skills I wouldn't learn in my family, so I sought out people who could teach me. One of the sources of support I explored was hypnotherapy, from which I learned the power of the subconscious mind. The subconscious mind stores all of your previous life experiences, beliefs, memories, skills, and situations you've been through and images you've seen.

Through hypnotherapy, it is possible to reprogram the messages the subconscious mind sends to the conscious self. I learned early in my exploration of hypnotherapy that if I didn't examine my deeply held beliefs, I would keep falling into self-harmful patterns. The main self-harmful pattern I dealt with was harsh self-talk. I told myself I was worthless and not doing anything good with my life. I suspect I had this belief of worthlessness because, in my family, it wasn't okay to have any big, "negative" emotions like anger or grief.

Whenever I needed or wanted to cry, I was sent to my room to be alone. The same for expressions of anger. As a result, I spent a fair amount of time alone as a young child with big, all-body-consuming emotions. In those alone times, I told myself the story that I was worthless and that no one cared about me or my situation. I believed that since I was most often alone when having big, difficult emotions, that no one really cared or even knew that I was even alive. I began to believe that I was only valuable or worth anything if I was contributing to the lives of others. Paying attention to myself or my own needs was discouraged, and I internalized that belief.

One of the things I explored in hypnotherapy was how tired I felt much of the time. I realized I had learned from my parents that it was best to be busy all the time. Resting and relaxing were not encouraged in my family, and I had made that message mine. It took a while, but through hypnotherapy and regular talk therapy, I gradually learned it's OK to rest and relax. I slowed down. When I became an endurance athlete and learned about periodization, which is training in periods of time, I learned that two of the key periods are "rest days" and "off season," which is essentially weeks or months of rest days. I was grateful I had learned the value of down time.

Intrinsic motivation allows us to notice what drives us from the inside. I learned the value of allowing myself rest and relaxation time. I learned that I had more energy for the athletic events I loved to do when I listened to my wise Inner Healer, who at critical moments seemed to know when to push and when to rest. Take a moment and think about what your intrinsic motivations are. Breathe into this insight.

EXTRINSIC MOTIVATION

Extrinsic motivation comes from outside of you (external). There is a reward or approval from others for doing a task. This might be praise, money, an ego prize, or status. It's difficult to rely upon extrinsic motivation because it depends on factors outside us. As a result, this sort of motivation is much less durable or long-lasting. It can temporarily spur us to action but, once the incentive is removed, it can cause a big drop in motivation.

Extrinsic motivation can be handy at times. I find signing up for a race or athletic event very motivating. Signing up for a race makes it real and that causes me to backward plan my training. Meaning I figure out when the race will be, and then from that day backward to the day I signed up, I figure out how many weeks or months I have to get ready to compete.

Friends as Extrinsic Motivation

During the first year of the COVID-19 pandemic, all of my planned races got canceled. Signing up for a race counts as extrinsic motivation. Especially if you've done at least one race and you know how important it is to train for the race. Needless to say, when all the races I had signed up for got canceled and refunded, my motivation to keep active went down the drain. It was disheartening.

Thankfully, I am part of a casual triathlon group called Team Looking Sharp. Jenny and Brooke started this team after Jenny finished breast cancer treatments and they were out walking together. Jenny had just gotten an email from the YWCA Minneapolis Women's Triathlon and she suddenly thought to herself, *I should do this!* She mentioned it to Brooke and Brooke said, "Yes, let's do it." Jenny's husband, Bob, had given her a card when she was bald from chemo with an image of a hedgehog looking at itself in the mirror. The card said, "Looking Sharp!" This became their name because they wanted to look sharp as they looked in the mirror and at each other, and become triathletes.

That first year there were three of them on the team. As the years went by, they kept inviting other women to join. One year,

Brooke invited me to join. I'd been doing the YWCA Women's Tri for a few years, but I did it by myself. For a few years, my endocrinologist had a triathlon team that did this particular race. I had done the race for a few years with them, which was super fun. Other than my endocrinologist, however, I didn't become close with anyone who was on the team. Essentially, I felt pretty alone as a triathlete in the Twin Cities. Unlike my triathlon experience in Colorado, I hadn't connected with any triathletes in Minnesota. I knew there were others here, but I hadn't become friends with any of them. To be invited to join Brooke and Jenny and the others they recruited felt like a gift from the heavens.

As the years went by, I kept doing the triathlon and training with the women of Team Looking Sharp. Slowly and surely, I became close friends with many of these women. That happens when you start spending two to four days a week swimming, biking, and running (and during the winter, cross-country skiing) with people. Making friends as an adult isn't always easy, especially if you aren't married and don't have children, as is my case. Turns out making friends with fellow athletes is a wonderful way to make purposeful, joyful connections. Having friends makes motivation easier. Having a community to train with for your event bolsters the joy and pleasure in doing your sport, which bolsters intrinsic motivation. Then having friends you will do the race alongside makes the extrinsic motivation fresh and fun.

Along the way I continued to do self-healing work, which, it turns out, was critical to do. Because I held a deeply internalized belief that I wasn't worth anything, it was nearly impossible for me to believe that friends would stick by me. In fact, over the years I've lost countless friends. One life-altering example began when I created a company to help people with diabetes become endurance athletes, TeamWILD Athletics LLC. I have since learned that losing friends and gaining friends happens in life. Ups and downs of various heights happen to everyone, and the key is to not give up and to do what you need to in order to keep your motivation alive.

TEAMWILD

In the first year of TeamWILD, I gathered twenty women, three athletic coaches, and two medical people to train us to compete in the Austin, Texas, Half Ironman. The race took place on October 25, 2009. We lived all over the United States, although we did have a concentration of women and coaches in the Denver, Colorado, area where I lived at the time. These were the days before Zoom and easily accessible online courses, so our year of training primarily took place through emailing and team phone calls. We traveled to Austin together in April 2009 for a four-day training camp, where we started to get to know each other and solidify what we were going to do. We rented rooms in a local hotel, and we shared all our meals together. The laughter as we loaded our bikes to the trailer to go to the race venue and preview the route helped us bond.

Nearly all of the twenty of us doing the Half Ironman—a 1.2-mile swim, followed by a 56-mile bike and then a 13.1-mile run—were doing such an event for the first time. In addition to that, sixteen of the twenty of us had type 1 diabetes. It was a major undertaking. We accomplished the Half Ironman race with great success. All of us crossed the finish line!

FINANCIAL FAILURE

After the Half Ironman with TeamWILD, I started having trouble managing my financial life. I struggled to pay the people who were helping me to build the TeamWILD Athletics LLC business. I didn't know how to get help to sort out the financial aspects of running my own business. I was two years behind in paying my taxes in full. I had filed on time, and I was on a payment plan with the IRS, but I didn't know how I would ever pay them back. I felt very alone and very overwhelmed. I didn't tell anyone, since I felt like I should somehow already know how to fix things.

Remember, I'm the oldest child in my family, and I had already survived two rounds of breast cancer. At this point I had been successfully living with type 1 diabetes for more than thirty years. I felt responsible for everyone and everything around me. This made asking for help with my business extremely difficult. I was so ashamed I didn't even tell my therapist about my struggles. It was a deeply held belief that I was supposed to figure it out by reading books and being smart. Riding my bike and going for runs were the two things that kept me from completely giving up. I kept digging inside myself for motivation to keep going.

The tension got worse as 2012 started. Without telling anyone, I took out money from one of my retirement accounts to pay a few of the people who continued to create programs with me for TeamWILD. The sense of isolation increased. I had ended my relationship with my then-boyfriend and that created an even greater sense of aloneness.

The tax debt situation didn't improve; in fact, it got worse. TeamWILD wasn't making money, despite being popular

EXTREME HEALING

with everyone we told about it. I kept giving away programs, hoping that if enough people understood what an online training program was, it would catch on. We were ahead of the online training boom. In early June, it reached a head. I felt completely desperate. I was a total business failure. I felt utterly alone. The business financial failure piece overshadowed any sense of success I may have felt. I had no more internal motivation left. My sense of connection externally was difficult, if not impossible for me to sense. It was there, I learned later, but I was in so much despair that I couldn't feel it.

One day it got so bad, I decided the best way to handle it would be to leave. Meaning to leave this life. Worthlessness flooded my entire being. As a result, like when I was a child alone with big emotions in my body, I didn't think that anyone really noticed me.

NO MOTIVATION

I know now that very old (from my childhood) belief of thinking that no one noticed me is not accurate; but at that point in my life, I did not understand that. I was still caught in the sense that I didn't make a difference, that I wasn't noticed. I was profoundly ashamed of my financial failure. I was ashamed of my inability to figure out how to make enough money to support the business I had created and was very passionate about. Shame can be a debilitating emotion. If you notice you have shame choking you, please, please, please find help. Name it and find support.

The sense of feeling incapable and alone were so profound, I figured that it would be better to simply leave. I now know that many of us have felt this level of hopelessness, aloneness, and shame.

Part of the conundrum of feeling so alone is that it's impossible to realize we are never worthless, and we are always connected. I lost hope and I didn't see or understand that there was a web of support available to me. I offer my story as a reminder that you *do* matter and your well-being is important. If no one else feels available to you, please reach out to me. I will help you find your community. I will sit with you and hold space for where you are.

At the time, I figured my leaving would take me out of the equation, and then the IRS would have no one else to come after for my back taxes. If I was gone, then that debt would be gone. Plus, if I were dead, then I wouldn't need any retirement money. Not an ideal retirement strategy, I've learned.

Additionally, I profoundly believed that people didn't really notice or care about me. I figured since our TeamWILD programs were barely selling, what I had to contribute to the world wasn't worth continuing to live for.

On June 11, 2012, I took a few sleeping pills, and I took an excess of insulin. I went out to my backyard, and I fell asleep on the lawn. I am not sure how long I slept. Somewhat miraculously, I did wake up. When I woke up, I was crying and I realized I wasn't quite ready to go. I made a vow that later, if I couldn't figure out my situation, I would try again. I remember, very dimly, deciding to give myself one year to see if I could sort out my situation. If I couldn't, then I would leave in one year.

On that day in 2012, I'm not sure how I got help. I do know that I did get some help. I reached out. My old boyfriend came and stayed with me for almost a month. We hosted

CampWILD, and I attended and led. I went back to therapy. The irony is that I *still* never told anyone just how financially overwhelmed I was, how lost I felt about how to figure out managing the business I oversaw. I continued to keep that desperation close in, not baring my truth to anyone. I was skimming around the truth. I still hoped that I would and thought that I should somehow figure it out by myself.

I decided to leave Colorado. I thought being closer to my mother and brother and his family would be a helpful thing. I hoped that would help with the aloneness and isolation I felt. The idea was that for a few months, while my house in Colorado was on the market, I would live with my mom. Turns out that was not a good decision. My mom hated living with my dog (too much shedding). I found myself vacuuming every other day and sweeping the floors every day. Still not to satisfaction.

Plus, I noticed that I couldn't read my mother. I couldn't figure out if she was open to talking, if she wanted to eat together, or not. I generally felt like I was massively in her way. I've lived with lots of housemates over the years, and often I'm the one who convenes house meetings. I couldn't figure out how to have a purposeful conversation about living together. After about one month, I found a little unit a few miles away, in a trendy, welcoming Minneapolis neighborhood.

During this time, I was still attempting to make a living with TeamWILD. Additionally, I was doing some speaking and coaching engagements with the American Diabetes Association Tour de Cure bicycle rides. They paid me a small amount of money for those engagements. I was eking out a barely livable income, just enough for rent, food, and to keep my car running. It was a month-to-month challenge, and the financial desperation grew.

I revealed some of my challenges with the IRS to my mother. She did offer to help me sort some of it out. I remember we went to a tax lawyer. The meeting was overwhelming and not helpful. Both of us were disappointed. I realized my mother didn't really understand the mess I was in. She had never been a business owner. I stopped talking with her about the challenges I was feeling or facing in regard to my financial difficulty. My isolation with my financial problem started to escalate.

In early 2013, the IRS started coming after me with intensity. At first I ignored them, hoping they would go away. They didn't. Finally, after yet another IRS letter in late April, I tried calling the agent who had sent the letter. That agent was not in on the day I called. The person I talked to didn't understand my case, except to tell me I owed a lot of money, and I had better pay as much as I could as quickly as I could. I got off the phone feeling completely destitute.

That spring, the TeamWILD working group was working hard to recruit people to CampWILD, a training camp for adults with diabetes to work on their athletic knowledge and skills. I felt the need to remain optimistic and upbeat. Again, I did not tell any of the working group just how overwhelmed and desperate I was feeling. I kept my pain and confusion to myself. I believed I was supposed to be the strong one. In essence, I didn't trust anyone.

In early June 2013, I went to Chicago for their American Diabetes Association Tour de Cure bike ride. It was a wonderful ride. Their organizing volunteers were very welcoming and friendly. Sadly, at that point, I felt more and more distant from everyone and everything. Some part of me knew that I was nearing my one-year deadline for figuring things out. Essentially, I had *not* figured anything out.

I did not feel connected to people. I felt more distant, more isolated. I was often in a dissociated state. Dissociation is a coping mechanism where the mind and the body disconnect. In my case, I can lose time, I have gaps in my memory, and I often don't feel real. Despite having found a Minnesota therapist, I had not revealed my desperate financial situation or my intense isolation to this person. I had perfected the ability to project a put-together life. I don't suffer from depression, and I was still doing social things with people, and I still hoped that miraculously I would somehow, without getting any actual help, figure out my dire financial situation with the IRS.

TIME'S UP

I don't remember writing a suicide note, but I did write one. I left it on my desk in my apartment. I made arrangements with my landlord to take care of my dog. I don't know what I told them. I left my phone in my apartment. I was serious about following through with my decision to leave, to die. I couldn't find a solution to my crisis. I wasn't smart enough. I wasn't connected enough. Essentially, I believed no one would notice I was gone. I believed that people would simply carry on, most likely better without me in the picture.

I realize now that belonging and being connected were not things I felt as a child. Given the trauma I grew up with, sexual abuse by my father, my maternal grandfather, and a babysitter, I figured out as a child that love was conditional. It was my job to tune into what would cause danger and hurt to happen, so as to avoid pain. I learned early that the only person I could trust was myself. It was a lonely childhood.

I learned I had to be completely self-reliant. I did not learn or experience how to feel connected to a community. I had not ever revealed my complete isolation. Like I mentioned earlier, I am the oldest, and as the oldest, I felt responsible. In this instance, I felt protective of my family. I wanted to preserve the myth that my family was perfect.

I figured, since I was clearly *not* perfect, especially in regard to financial management, then I should exit the scene. I believed that it would be better for me to die by suicide than to cause public embarrassment for my financial failure. I was convinced that would be a better option.

I took matters into my hands again on June 11, 2013. I shifted into a completely dissociated place. I don't remember giving myself a massive overdose of insulin, and I don't remember taking over half a bottle of sleeping pills—I did both. Somehow, I managed to drive myself away from where I lived, to a random, rarely used road in Edina, Minnesota.

I went missing for three days. During that time, a few things happened that I don't fully understand to this day. My family figured out that I was missing first. My sister-in-law posted something to my Facebook page, asking if anyone had seen me. That resulted in a small group of people I knew from the Tour de Cure Twin Cities to create an extensive search for me.

Their search extended to Denver, Colorado, and to Santa Cruz, California, both cities where I had lived for more than nine years each. In addition, in the months before I went missing, several women had been randomly raped, so my being missing caught the attention of the Twin Cities media. As a result, for the days I was missing, people searched methodically for me all over the Minneapolis–Saint Paul, Minnesota, area.

I was found by a random man who lived near where my car was parked. He had seen my car in the morning when he was out for a walk. Then when he got home from work he took another walk and he again saw my car. He thought it was unusual that the same car would be in the same place both in the morning and the early evening. He approached my car to see if he could see anything inside the car. He saw me in a reclining position in the driver's seat. He had not heard about me being missing, but he knew he should call for help, so he called the police.

When the police got there, they broke open the car. Apparently, the inside of the car was over 112 degrees, yes, it was *hot*. They got me into an ambulance, and they took me to the hospital. I remained in a coma for two more days, during which time they tested me for all the possible drugs I could have taken.

After a few days, I started to come out of the coma. I don't remember waking up, but slowly I did. The hospital then moved me to the psychiatric ward, where I stayed for another thirty-two days. It was unclear how extensive the damage was to my brain or my well-being. I couldn't speak clearly, and I couldn't function normally.

What I do remember was that I knew I was okay being alive. In fact, I remember that one of my first thoughts was that there was more that I needed to do with this life. I hadn't yet remembered my near-death experience, I just knew I wasn't dead for a reason.

RECONNECTION

At first, in the psychiatric ward, they didn't have anyone else with a similar situation and, as a result, they didn't know how to deal with me. I had forgotten how to do things like fetch my food from the trays they brought to feed us. I didn't know how to take a shower. I was lost. I was very quiet, as I couldn't remember how to form words.

I had been a long-time meditator, and I remembered how to sit in meditation. Very quickly, I realized that meditating every day was a good way to spend time. All I did was sit upright in a lotus position on a towel up against the wall in my room. I focused hour after hour on my breathing. I observed my thoughts but didn't attach myself to them. As I sat breathing quietly, I noticed that I spiritually felt connected to the bigger world.

No one came to visit me. I didn't catch on to why no one came to see me. I just noticed that every single other person who was on the ward had regular visitors. No visitors fed my belief that no one noticed me or cared if I was alive or dead. What I didn't understand until much later was that my family told the wide community of more than 800 people who had created a special Facebook group about me that people were directed to "leave me and my family alone."

I am thankful that after more than three weeks at the hospital, my longtime triathlon friend Delinda from Colorado decided to come visit me, defying the directive from my biological family members. Seeing Delinda was like a fresh breeze of affirmation. We hugged hello and Delinda told me how glad she was to see me and know that I was recovering. She asked thoughtful, kind questions. She told me that there were people in the world that cared about my well-being and that wanted to know how I was doing. It was refreshing and rejuvenating to begin to connect with the circle of friends who cared about me.

Ironically, my mother didn't come very often to see me. My sister had come to Minnesota to help at the time I was first missing, and she was there at the very start of me being in the coma in the hospital, but then she went back to Oregon and didn't communicate with me anymore. My brother and his family didn't come to see me that I can remember, except once. My biological family told people to leave me alone, and then they themselves also left me alone.

My first clear memory happened the day that my mother came to see me. She had brought with her a folder. The folder contained various expenses I had, such as car insurance and other bills. What I vividly recall is that as she sat in a chair in the locked facility where my bed was. She told me that she thought my life was a complete mess. She had no idea how I would ever get my life in financial order again. She then proceeded to tell me that she thought I was a total failure, and that she didn't know how I would ever sort things out.

Her words registered.

In response, I felt a part of my brain come alive again. Something shook inside of me. I remember taking a deep breath and looking at her and asking her, "Do you know what you are saying to me?" She replied that yes, she knew what she was saying.

I then said, "I am not dead. I came to the realization that I want to live. I have more to do in this life, and to do those things, I need to have only those people around me who believe in me and my ability to survive and sort things out. It sounds like you don't believe in me." What I remember is that she agreed, she did not believe in me. I said to her that if she wasn't going to be on my team, she needed to leave immediately.

She got up and left. That was the last time I had a meaningful conversation with my mother.

Slowly I regained brain function. The four to six hours of meditation I did every day helped my brain recover. I became a witness to my thoughts, which allowed the neural pathways in my damaged brain to heal. I figured out how to use the one computer available to all of us on the ward, even though we were only allowed access for fifteen minutes at a time. I remember the first time I went on Facebook while in the hospital. I was astonished at the amount of support that was out there for me.

The one saving grace that happened while I was in that psychiatric ward was meeting the endocrinologist they assigned to help with my diabetes. Her name is Rebecca Mattison.[1] She was the one kind, reliable person I met during that "more than one month" stay in the hospital. She figured out quickly that I wasn't massively depressed like the hospital psychiatrist insisted. She knew there was more to my story than met the eye. She expressed interest in who I was. She recognized that I was grateful to still be alive, and that I wasn't suicidal any longer. Dr. Mattison continues to be the endocrinologist I see to help me navigate my diabetes care.

Eventually they let me out of the hospital. I went back to my apartment, but was shortly after forced to find a new place to live. Thanks to a connection I had made at the meditation center I attended, I found a new place to live fairly easily and my friend and diabetes superstar Scott Johnson[2] helped me make the move.

A Minneapolis social worker helped me get food stamps and apply for and receive monthly emergency funding. This helped me for more than two years as I regained my brain function and my financial footing. Additionally, those 800 Facebook friends had raised money that I proceeded to live on for the next year.

I attended an outpatient mental health clinic every day for eight weeks. At this clinic, I met a psychiatrist who said that it did not seem like I was depressed. Her diagnosis was post-traumatic stress disorder, PTSD, given all that I had endured from childhood on. The moment she told me that, I burst into tears.

For the first time, a mental health diagnosis made sense to me. I wasn't depressed; instead I suffered from PTSD. Some people who suffer from PTSD have depression also, and some of us don't. Post-traumatic stress syndrome happens to some people when they witness or experience a traumatic event. In my case, it was the repeated sexual abuse of my childhood in combination with witnessing the repeated low blood sugar, almost death events that my father experienced through my childhood and youth. To add more to the mix, when I was a freshman in college, I was raped by another college student who lived in my dorm. I thought it was my fault that he did that, a common thing for a victim of childhood abuse to think when an event repeats itself in adulthood. Please see the resources at the end of this chapter to learn more about PTSD.

Slowly, step by step, I rebuilt my life. In the years since this happened, I have gotten amazing support and help. I decided to finally tell my truth to the therapists I was seeing. In being vulnerable with telling my truth, I got the help I had longed for my whole life.

I got financial help. I filed bankruptcy. I got financial coaching, which led to becoming a financial coach. I found a job that I love. I learned how to live within my means. I continue to meditate every day. I forgive myself every day for not being perfect. I have almost no contact with most of my biological family. A few of them dislike me quite a bit.

I am learning to be close to people. I have a circle of beloved friends and colleagues. I have come to believe (and feel in my bones and in my heart as well as my head) that I do matter. I do belong. This insight was hard won. It has taken much deep introspection to learn how to mother and father myself, and to see that I do have an impact. My being dead by my own hand wasn't and isn't the better option. I have survived the shame of financial failure. I still belong. There is support and help in the world for me. And for you.

There is help for all of us. Breathe into that.

NEW BEGINNINGS

The closing of TeamWILD, along with my suicide attempts, resulted in the ending of nearly all the friendships I had made through TeamWILD. It took me a few years to realize that happened largely due to not believing I was good enough or worthy of love or friendship. I didn't know how to be vulnerable and trusting with the people around me.

The loss of the friendships with the more than nine women who were the early athletes and coaches of TeamWILD still haunts me. In the present day, it reminds me to slow down and notice if I'm trying to control a situation. And if I am, I consciously breathe into letting go, and remind myself that as an adult I am safe and I do belong, simply because I exist.

When I see these nine women on Facebook or other social media platforms, and I see their continued connection with one another, I breathe deeply, and I send them well wishes, and I again let go. I remind myself I am a good friend and I have found good people with whom to exercise, enter races, and have athletic fun. I didn't know how to connect in an authentic way back then. I have learned how to be in connection and community, and now I am connected.

I know some of you have had big failures and big despair in your life. These failures and this despair can cause your motivation to go out the window. You might wonder if you will ever again care about your physical well-being. I am here to tell you that you can find your way again. Please, be gentle and kind to yourself. Most important, find people to hold space for you.

UNDERSTAND YOURSELF

Athletically, it pays off to take time to examine where your motivation comes from. My decision to do The Bicycle Tour of Colorado when I was thirty-nine stemmed from a deep internal drive to find out if I was strong enough to take on and complete such a challenge. Could I figure out my diabetes well enough to manage such an adventure? Later, a week after finishing radiation therapy, I wondered if I could do my first triathlon. Both challenges came from an internal motivation to discover what I was capable of. I was intrinsically motivated.

I discovered that extrinsic motivation spoke to me as well. I enjoyed the applause and compliments I got upon completing these athletic events. Knowing that the celebration, even the status, would come as a result of doing long-distance athletic events kept me going and signing up for more. Often there's a beautiful mix of both internal and external motivation. This causes me to circle back to the idea of inspiration.

Technically, motivation and inspiration are interchangeable. However, I experience these two concepts in different ways. Motivation feels like drive or action. Inspiration causes me to breathe deeply, to choose to bring something into my body and spirit. Motivation causes me to move. Inspiration touches my heart, which in a roundabout way will often morph into motivation.

A few months before the pandemic hit, I joined a running club called Run Minnesota. They specialize in distance running. Joining this group motivated me to consider doing another 10-mile running race. One of the men in the group, Mike, is an older runner; he was nearing seventy when I met him. He was training for a half marathon. He has a full head of white hair, and he's quite a fast runner. Seeing his enthusiasm, sense of dedication, and fun touched my heart and caused me to visualize myself at his age, continuing to be a runner in good health and fitness. That inspiration solidified my desire to become a year-round runner.

INSPIRATION

There are days when I lack the inspiration or the motivation to get moving. Meaning, when I wake up, I don't have energy or drive to get up and get to the planned exercise for the day. What I do now is notice my lack of energy and desire, observing it as if from a small distance away. Then I take a deep breath and I go into my meditation practice. I use a few different meditation apps these days. My favorite is the free Insight Timer app[3] that I have on my phone. On days when I notice my resistance to exercise, I choose meditations related to the body.

The act of rhythmic, focused breathing causes me to come back into my body, accepting whatever is happening in this moment. Given my experience with dissociation, this skill of coming back into my body with meditation is helpful. By paying close attention in this way, what happens is I settle. I remember that nearly every time I do the exercise I have planned, I end up with more energy. This pause calls me back to a truth that then causes me to practically leap out of bed ready to put on my exercise clothes and get to it.

MEDITATION AND INSPIRATION

I've attended several week-long meditation retreats. One of my early meditation instructors is the renowned meditation teacher Jack Kornfield, cofounder of the Insight Meditation Society and one of the first westerners to make meditation accessible to those in the western world.

On one of my first meditation retreats, we were asked to be in silence for a whole day, one of the hardest requests ever made of me. The request was to sit in meditation and to eat our meals in silence and to do everything for the entire day in complete silence. As I mentioned earlier, I was distancing myself from my body to escape feeling its pain and had learned to talk constantly, to not be in my own inner truth.

Early in my teaching career, I became friends with a young man named Rama. One day we were in my car driving home from an event and Rama turned to me and he said, "Mari, please stop talking. Let's just be here in this space together." I was confused. I asked him what he meant, of course. "Mari, you talk all the time. You barely pause. If ever there's an empty space between us, you immediately fill it with words. I've noticed you do this with nearly everyone you know. Why do you want to fill all the empty space? What would happen if you slowed down and enjoyed the silence?" This was the first time anyone pointed out to me my incessant talking.

When my teacher Jack asked us to spend a day in silence, terror filled my body. As I continued my inner healing work, I learned that I was detached from quite a bit of who I was, having learned to keep busy and keep talking as avoidance strategies. Getting quiet and focusing on my breath took courage.

I didn't succeed that first day at the meditation retreat. I found the talkers at a lunch table and was relieved to have a chat with a small group. Luckily, Jack knew how hard it was for some of us to be silent. Without judgment, when we all returned to the meditation hall, he invited us back to the breath and to silence. He reassured us that it was OK to allow whatever emotions to arise, to give them space. That made sense, even if it was uncomfortable at times.

It was at one of these meditation/breathwork retreats that I met my dear friend Chris Klebl, who I told you about in chapter one. He's the person who sat up so tall and present. Just noticing Chris sitting so tall in the meditation hall inspired me to sit up straighter and go inside to hear what wanted to be heard. This early meditation training practice served me well when I was in that psychiatric hospital. It is a practice that continues to serve me. I highly recommend mindfulness meditation. It will help you with inspiration and motivation, critical things for athletic success.

INSPIRATION TO GET STARTED
AND TO SLOW DOWN

Simply inhaling and noticing the mind and body allows me to take action. Inhaling is inspiration. Conscious breathing inspires me. I know, it seems simple, and it is. Try it.

Because I grew up believing that my value was related to how busy and productive I was in the world, slowing down is not easy for me. I've been able to do a lot of therapy. I've had many opportunities in which people reflected me to myself and held space for me to slow down and reflect on why I have the beliefs I have. With repeated practice doing this over and over again, these experiences have resulted in learning the power and value of simply taking a deep breath and giving myself a minute or two to simply slow down and tune into what is happening in my body and mind.

I've learned the value of feeling joy, sadness, confusion, happiness, inspiration, or motivation as it is living in my body. Taking the time to slow down, take a breath, and tune into my heart or my stomach or perhaps a spot in my neck—to notice the emotions that are in my body—has taught me quite a bit about the wisdom *of* my body and *in* my body. Slowing down has taught me, by example, that emotions really do live in the body.

Recently I was out on a five-mile run alongside the frozen Mississippi River by myself. I left my headset turned off and I focused on my breathing. It was about 12 degrees Fahrenheit and that didn't include the windchill. It took me about fifteen minutes to warm up and once I was done shivering, I tuned into my body. I had lifted weights the day before and my legs and butt were sore from the squats, lunges, and one-legged hip sled exercises I had done. I breathed deeply and asked my body how it was doing.

It spoke to me in swatches of color, meaning despite the gray and white of the cloudy cold day there were images in my mind of bright blues, yellows, oranges, and greens. Hopeful, powerful colors. I felt emotions of optimism, courage, strength, and hope flow through my being. The soreness in my body was helping me get faster and stronger as a runner. The sense was that the sore would fade. It was okay to feel the soreness, not avoid it, as I ran. Despite the minor pain I felt and the tiredness, I was glad I had gotten out for this run on this cold, dreary day. As I tuned into my body and my emotions as I ran, I found myself feeling grateful I was out running. Grateful I could run, and already thinking about my next run.

On those days I feel too busy or distracted to exercise, I've learned a few things that help. I set myself up for success. Turns out these steps are similar to what James Clear teaches in his book *Atomic Habits: An Easy and Proven Way to Build Good Habits and Break Bad Ones.*[4] All of these ways break down the step to short, easily accomplished steps to make taking action nearly effortless. Turns out we are creatures who prefer the easiest way to get something done.

I offer these five ways to you to help you get inspired and motivated to get yourself out there and move your beautiful body.

FIVE WAYS TO GET OUT THE DOOR

1: Have your gear clean and easily accessible.

I always have a gym bag ready to go. I store my gym bag in a highly visible spot in my bedroom. My gym bag is a backpack that is bright orange, so it catches my eye and reminds me to think about when I'm next going to the gym. In it, I have clean workout clothes right down to the socks, plus a towel and shampoo. Since I have diabetes, I also have glucose tabs packed in the bag and a few granola bars. I even keep a filled water bottle in the bag. At a moment's notice I can dash to the gym.

2: Get dressed to exercise, then decide.

On the days when, no matter what, I don't want to exercise, I break it down into the smallest steps possible. I don't say I'm going to the gym or for a walk or a run; I simply put on my workout clothes. Once I have the clothing on, it's easier to say, "OK, I'll walk out the door and then decide." Often, by this point, it's easier to just do it than not.

In the winter, I really break things down and talk to myself quite a bit. I tell myself to first find my cross-country skis. Then, I tell myself to find my snow pants, coat, hat, neck gaiter, and mittens. Then I put all the clothing on. THEN I decide if I will go outside and ski. As you might expect, I most often go skiing and have a great time doing it. And yes, I laugh quite a bit at myself.

3: Schedule workouts, even with yourself; keep the dates and celebrate.

I put all my workouts in my calendar with buzzer reminders. I have several Google calendars, one of which is specifically for my workouts. Every Sunday afternoon or early evening, I sit down with my calendar and schedule my exercise sessions for the week. I review my training calendar, and I spend at least three minutes visualizing the goal/event I'm training for.

This makes sure I'm prioritizing my exercise sessions. When I finish the session, I go back into my calendar where I jot down notes about the session, including how many miles or yards (in the case of swimming) I did. I also put an X and an exclamation point in front of the name of the session. That way when I review my calendar, I can see how many sessions I completed and how many miles I ran or biked or swam that week. It makes the celebration that much sweeter.

4: Schedule workouts with friends who will hold you accountable.

Having accountability partners makes a huge difference. Once, when I was training for a 100-mile bike ride, I had to do months of indoor bike training because there was too much snow to ride outdoors. So far, I am not a winter cyclist. There were six of us training for the 100-mile bike ride and we texted and called each other almost every Sunday to check in with each other about the rides we would do each week. Knowing this group valued training as much as I did made me want to do all my alone sessions and our group sessions.

5: Practice, practice, practice.

You've got your event scheduled. You have your gear. You have a training plan. You know a bit about nutrition. You have your supporters lined up, including training partners, family and friend spectators to cheer at your event, and your physical and mental care teams to help you manage your various health challenges.

Now what?

By reminding myself that it is practice, I don't have to be the fastest or the most skilled or the best: All that's required of me is to be out there doing the sport. That relieves a huge amount of pressure. The only thing I need to do is keep moving my body.

Heading out for a run or bike ride, I tell myself that it is practice. I do this because, perhaps like you, I like to be perfect and do things correctly. Relieving the need to be fast or perfect allows me to find my motivation when it skirts out of sight.

INSPIRATIONAL PEOPLE FOR MOMENTS OF WANTING TO GIVE UP

Terry Fox[5] is a Canadian man who at age eighteen was diagnosed with bone cancer in his leg. He had his leg amputated six inches above his knee. While he was in the hospital, he learned of another amputee runner. Very soon, he decided to run coast to coast in Canada, calling it his Marathon of Hope. He began training and, after eighteen months and 3,107 miles of training runs (all of them with his artificial leg), he began his Marathon of Hope by dipping his artificial leg in the Atlantic Ocean.

On average, Terry ran 26 miles a day for 143 days and covered 3,339 miles. He gathered a huge amount of media attention and support. I remember learning about Terry when I was learning how to run. I was profoundly inspired by how, despite the pain, Terry would look ahead to a stop sign or a tree and mentally he would tell himself to run just that far. When he got to the stop sign or tree, he would look ahead and pick the next landmark. He would break up a long, long run into tiny, bite-sized pieces and conquer one bite at a time.

Terry had to stop before reaching the Pacific coast because the cancer came back in his lungs. He had to stop and go home to battle it. He never did finish that run, dying just one month shy of his twenty-third birthday. Since then, more than $850 million Canadian has been raised for cancer research in Terry Fox's name. Runs are held in his honor worldwide.

There are times when I go out for a run, and I think of Terry Fox. I break the run into small bits, and I think of what he did for cancer research. When he was recovering from his amputation, he was in the hospital with many children who had cancer and he vowed that he would not forget their pain and suffering. He vowed to raise money for more research and he vowed to create more awareness. Before and after his death, this is exactly what he did. This inspirational life helps move me from inspiration to motivation to get outside and onto my bike, into my swimsuit, or in my run shoes.

You too can find motivation, both intrinsic and extrinsic. Along the way, pay attention to what inspires you. Notice what speaks to your heart. Use all that you can to get yourself out the door, and moving your beautiful body. I believe in you!

 TRY THIS

Journal

Get out your Athlete Journal and make yourself a few lists.

List 1: What are the internal motivators in your athletic life? Think about what brings you joy. Is it the feeling of being outside with the sun and wind and trees? Is it the delight of moving your body? Be specific and let yourself visualize and feel the joy as you imagine your internal motivators.

List 2: What are the external motivators in your athletic life?
Get as specific as you can. Consider some of the following: signing up for races, getting race gear, the prestige of being able to tell people you accomplished an athletic goal, getting a race medal to hang up where you see it to remind yourself of what you are capable of doing, and so much more. Let your imagination have fun!

List 3: What or who inspires you?
In particular, what things athletically inspire you? You can be as general or as specific as suits your fancy. Terry Fox regularly inspires me when I am dreading a long run. Use this list of inspiring people to motivate you.

If any of these lists intimidate you, write about what it is that intimidates you. Breathe deeply and go back in the chapter to the definitions of intrinsic and extrinsic motivation, and reflect on when in your life you've found intrinsic and extrinsic motivation that got you to take action.

If needed, also go back to chapter 3 and work more on your fears and obstacles. Remember, becoming an endurance athlete is not a linear path. It's much more of a spiral. It's okay to circle back when needed.

Notes

1.   See Rebecca Mattison, MD, at https://endoclinic.net.
2.   See Scott Johnson at https://scottsdiabetes.com.
3.   Find the Insight Timer meditation app at https://insighttimer.com.
4.   James Clear, *Atomic Habits: An Easy Proven Way to Build Good Habits & Break Bad Ones* (Avery, 2018), https://jamesclear.com.

5.   See Terry Fox at https://terryfox.org.

Resources

Hypnotherapy https://www.psychologytoday.com/us/therapy-types
/hypnotherapy

Mantras, https://chopra.com/articles/what-is-a-mantra

PTSD Resources: https://www.nami.org/About-Mental-Illness/Mental
-Health-Conditions/Posttraumatic-Stress-Disorder

Insight Meditation Society, https://www.dharma.org

Jack Kornfield, https://jackkornfield.com

CHAPTER 5

LEVEL UP BY SIGNING UP

"I have been impressed with the urgency of doing. Knowing is not enough; we must apply. Being willing is not enough; we must do."

—*LEONARDO DA VINCI*

I'VE NEVER BEEN A FAN OF WATCHING SPORTS ON TELEVISION. When I was a high school assistant principal, I supervised countless high school football, volleyball, basketball, baseball, and soccer games. Even though I knew most of the players, I preferred socializing at the games rather than watching the athletic action. That lack of spectating enthusiasm completely changed in July 2000 when my Paralympic athlete boyfriend, Chris, introduced me to the Tour de France, the professional bicycling race held every summer in France. The best male cyclists in the world race for three weeks, covering long distances almost every day for twenty-one days.

I was instantly mesmerized, watching every day, sometimes both the morning broadcast and the evening. I learned the names and histories of every cyclist. I was fascinated by the strategies used by the climbers and the sprinters. I was amazed at the capacity the cyclists had for suffering. Seeing American cyclist Tyler Hamilton ride with what ended up being a broken collarbone for days was astonishing. I began to wonder, *"What is my capacity to suffer?"*

When I was thirty-eight, I decided to learn more about my suffering capacity by doing The Bicycle Tour of Colorado, a 400-mile bike ride around Colorado. Two of the six days covered 100-mile routes and a lot of up and down steep mountain riding. I signed up for the ride a year in advance, my first step being to commit. Paying money for the event made my commitment real.

That's what I invite you to do in this chapter—sign up for an athletic event or race. It's time to make your commitment real.

WHEN THE FEAR LOOP STRIKES AGAIN

When you're in the fear loop, you are in the Stage of Change phase known as Pre-Contemplation, which is where there's no intention and little to no awareness that change would be helpful. Learning this helped me see how self-harmful the fear loop is for me.

I was solidly in the fear loop in the weeks before I signed up for The Bicycle Tour of Colorado. I wasn't sure I would belong, and I didn't have any friends who were doing the event. I kept telling myself that such a big athletic challenge was way beyond my skill and experience. I could have stayed in this place. Not taking on a big athletic challenge was my norm, so it was comfortable. Then, over a series of morning meditations, I kept hearing my inner voice telling me to try it. As I listened in nonjudgment to this voice, I slowly moved from Pre-Contemplation to Contemplation. It was a relief to get out of that fear loop.

Having no clue how to prepare athletically or diabetes-wise for such a ride, I sat down and outlined what I was willing to do, and from whom I would need to ask for guidance so I could do the ride.

I had attended a conference by the Diabetes Exercise Sports Association (or DESA, which no longer exists) in Chicago and heard an amazing endocrinologist, Dr. Matthew Corcoran,[1] speak about type 1 diabetes and endurance exercise. His insight and wisdom touched me. His approachable way included presentations that featured case studies of real people with diabetes who took on major physical challenges like marathons and long triathlons. He spoke about these athletes as people first, and people with diabetes second. I approached Dr. Matt and asked him if he would be willing to be my endocrinologist even though I lived in Denver, and he was in Chicago. Without a moment's hesitation he said, "Sure!" At the time I worked as a school development coach and two of my schools were in Chicago, so I combined seeing Dr. Matt with work visits to the city. We also emailed blood sugar information, insulin intake numbers, questions, and insights back and forth.

I asked cycling coach Nicole Freedman if she'd be willing to take me on as a client and devise a training plan to get me ready for seven continuous days of long-distance cycling. As Dr. Matt had done, Nicole said, "For sure! Let's do this!" Turns out she'd always wanted to learn more about diabetes. When you're ready for support, and you take that first tiny step of declaring your intention, your teachers and guides arrive. I have found this to be true over and over again.

The first thing Nicole had me do was take my LeMond Zurich road bike to the bike shop for a complete tune-up. Trusting your gear is a vital first step. I also had an official bike fit. Making sure the bike fits you is critical for comfort for long hours of riding. In chapter 8, I go into detail about the importance of gear.

DIABETES ON THE BIKE

Dr. Matt and I experimented with not lowering my basal rate (which is the background insulin being delivered by my insulin pump) while I was riding and using the basal insulin to cover the carbohydrates I needed to eat every hour to maintain the glucose levels I needed for performance. It was from Nicole, who does not have diabetes, that I learned that it was essential to eat as I was riding. Before meeting and working with Nicole, I made my nutrition decisions based on what my blood sugar was doing. Nicole convinced me I needed to eat when I was doing long rides, no matter what my blood sugar was.

After much experimentation, we figured it out for my body. For those of you readers who have diabetes, you likely already know that diabetes is living with a constant science experiment. All that experimentation involved so much trial and error that there were days that it just felt like tremendous suffering, with no way out. As you know, there is physical suffering and there is mental suffering. Sometimes, it's difficult to tell the difference. I have a physical condition that technically and directly doesn't cause physical pain in my body most days. My body makes zero insulin so I have to inject (in my case via an insulin pump) the hormone insulin to manage the carbohydrates I consume.

I've worn an insulin pump for nearly thirty years and over the years I've learned to navigate the "every three days" jab of putting in a new infusion set, which requires putting a needle into my stomach, arm, or leg. That jab hardly ever physically hurts. However, there are times when the repetition and the forced need to change my infusion set mentally hurts. It's time I could have spent doing something much more enjoyable. Truth be told, nearly anything is more enjoyable than changing an insulin pump infusion set. Sometimes when I'm making the set change, I jab the site into a nerve ending and I yelp. The combo of mental exhaustion and physical pain is wearing.

I remember biking on days when the insulin strategy didn't provide me with enough insulin to cover the carbohydrates I was eating, and my blood sugar would go soaring up, sometimes into the 400s. For those of you that don't have diabetes, the ideal blood sugar for all of us is somewhere between 70 mg/dl and 110 mg/dl.

When my blood sugar skyrocketed, I felt horrible and, depending on where I was on a cycling route, my options would at times be limited. The version of horrible in my case is that my thinking can be disrupted. I am often super thirsty as my body is attempting to lower my blood sugar, which causes the kidneys to work overtime. At times, my vision can get blurry.

I learned that drinking straight water was extremely helpful. The water helped my kidneys flush the extra glucose out of my system. I also learned to take micro-boluses. A bolus is when insulin is given in a dose to cover the carbs eaten or to lower a high blood sugar. When the blood sugar goes high, there is a tendency to want to rage bolus. A rage bolus is when a person with diabetes takes as much insulin as possible, or more, to get the blood sugar down into a normal range as quickly as possible. A micro-bolus is when the person with diabetes takes half, or less, than the amount of insulin needed to get the blood sugar back in range. Taking a micro-bolus helps prevent low blood sugar as I keep moving my body on the bike. If I was far from home, out on my bike, I had to mentally figure out a way to keep riding. To keep riding while my blood sugar was far from ideal made me feel horrible and on the edge of panic.

MANTRAS FOR FOCUS

I learned the power of mantras for moments like this. I would take 50 percent of the bolus needed to get my blood sugar back into a normal range, get back on the bike, and start my mantra recitation. Over and over I would say to myself, "Dear Body, you have enough insulin. Cells, keep doing good work. Let the insulin and the movement get the insulin into the cells. You are strong. Relax. Trust. Keep pedaling. Enjoy this beautiful day. You are loved. You can do this. Keep pedaling."

In part because of my difficult childhood, knowing how to comfort myself was something I figured out how to do early. I didn't know that mantras of self-comfort and focus were what self-talk of encouragement were called. I just knew as a child that such self-talk felt good in my being. Turns out, as I was becoming an athlete, such self-talk is highly helpful. They say that what you say to yourself matters in how you show up in the world. As I was out on my bike with terrible blood sugars and feeling yucky, the mantras and positive self-talk kept me peddling and kept my anxiety to a minimum.

As you reflect on your physical challenges, start to consider what your mantras for support could be. Knowing what you can say to yourself when the going gets tough will help keep your anxiety down and your spirits high.

THE BICYCLE TOUR OF COLORADO

My first foray into "real" endurance athletics was the Bicycle Tour of Colorado. I put "real" in quotation marks because the ride introduced me to a whole new way of life, one characterized by the camaraderie of hundreds of people all doing the same athletic endeavor at the same time. I had never been a part of such a community. For the first time in my life, I felt like I had found my people. I belonged. Since I had rarely felt like I belonged anywhere and with anyone, this was a powerful, transformative experience.

Then there were the athletic aspects of the adventure, and the rhythm of life that were all new to me. We climbed more than 10,000 feet one day and, on two different days, rode 100 miles up and down the Rocky Mountains. We woke up early every day, packed our tents and gear, and hauled our things over to the trucks, who would bring our gear to the next town where we would sleep. We had breakfast, and then we clipped onto our bike pedals as the sun was rising.

TRAINING

The Bicycle Tour of Colorado started June 26, the anniversary of the day in 1981 on which I found out I had diabetes. What a perfect day to begin this challenging athletic undertaking (the most difficult physical event I'd ever attempted). I officially started my training program on the first of February, five and a half months before the ride, with no idea how much I would discover and learn. I just knew that I had set the goal, and I had lined up the perfect support in Dr. Matt and Coach Nicole.

Over the weeks and months, Nicole sent me training plans that had me training by hours of riding, rather than miles, which I loved. This method focused on time on the bike versus how fast I was covering miles. The idea behind this method is to log hours on the bike versus being hung up on miles ridden. This coaching method focuses on getting used to spending long hours on the bike in the saddle. Many long ride days, I was pleasantly surprised at how many miles I could cover in one session.

About a month and a half before the tour, I was riding fifteen to eighteen hours a week. This was in addition to my full-time job. Finding time to ride wasn't easy, but I had my big hairy audacious goal (BHAG)[2] in mind and that was enough to get me out of bed early to start work early, giving me three or four hours of daylight at workday's end to get on my bike and ride.

Nicole had me doing all kinds of drills on the bike, including a one-legged drill where you unclip one bike shoe and pedal with just one leg for a minute at a time and then switch legs. Sounds easy, but it isn't. Turns out our bodies seamlessly compensate for our weaknesses. When you isolate a part of your body, you discover weaknesses previously undetectable. By doing one-legged drills, I built up my weaker leg, which in my case is my left leg, which made my whole body stronger. She also had me do all kinds of sprints and time myself going up mountains. Nicole as a coach brought countless insights to my training, her knowledge being so much greater than my own. She broke her wealth of knowledge down into bite-sized bits that I could incorporate slowly and surely. Having a coach by your side as you undertake an athletic challenge is priceless.

I rarely rode with anyone. At that point, I didn't really know any other cyclists in Denver. Granted, lots of cyclists live in Colorado; I just wasn't brave enough to join any cycling groups, so I rode alone. I was afraid I wouldn't be able to keep up with a group, or that I wouldn't have the correct gear, or that my bike wasn't good enough. In my imagined comparisons, I always came out on the "not good enough" side of the scale. This was a broken record from my childhood. I hadn't yet worked through all of these old fears and obstacles.

The routes were so beautiful that I never felt lonely. The mountains, trees, rivers, and birds reflected in the blue sky kept me company. Riding enhanced my communion with spirit and became a meditation. I had started a meditation practice years earlier but was new to moving meditation. As I rode along, paying attention to what was happening in my body, I learned to breathe deeply and carefully from the core of my body. I learned to feel the power in my legs and to trust how the bike felt underneath me. The hours and hours of riding taught me to be in the now, to let go of my worries, and feel my wholeness.

Finally, the training was done. A few days before the tour started, my friend Jeff brought over one of Lance Armstrong's yellow Livestrong wristbands. This was long before we knew about Lance's doping during the Tour de France. We admired him as an athlete who'd overcome cancer and helped bring a love of cycling to the United States. I loved the yellow bracelet, put it on and wore it the whole tour. It served as a visible reminder that I'd done the work and could tackle this monumental challenge.

I gathered my gear for the trip: a tent, a good sleeping bag, and a sleeping mat. I rounded up enough bike shorts, bike jerseys, bike socks, and rain gear for the week. I wouldn't have a washing machine, so having enough clothing was essential. I didn't know anyone who would be on the trip and was nervous about doing this all alone. Although taking on a big challenge alone can be a deterrent for many, I wasn't willing to let my lack of cycling friends keep me from accomplishing this BHAG I'd set for myself. Please start thinking about your BHAG.

I reminded myself often that doing this tour was important to me, although I didn't at the time know why. My inner wisdom knew I was an endurance road cyclist. I decided to trust that. With relative ease on the tour, I started to make cycling friends. I found people who rode at my speed and who asked me questions and shared their life stories with me. Riding and chatting with new people is fun, I discovered. Eating the food the ride provided for us was delicious. Turns out burning thousands of calories a day makes food taste extra good. There was lots of laughter. I was pleased that my ability to manage my insulin, food, and hydration and to keep my blood sugars in range during the ride was quite easy given how much experimentation and trial and error I had done in preparation. My hard work paid off, making the ride enjoyable. The other amazing surprise was that athletically, all the training I had done prepared me to climb up those big mountains with strength and confidence. At the end of every day, as I took a shower and went to bed early, I metaphorically patted myself on the back for how many hours I had put in, and how prepared my body was to accomplish this challenge.

Completing The Bicycle Tour of Colorado remains an accomplishment of which I'm very proud. Today, whenever I go on a long ride alone, I reflect on how much fun I had and how glorious it was to discover my endurance cycling passion.

THE CHALLENGE OF CANCER

When I finished the 400-mile bike ride across Colorado, I was joyously happy. I had made new friends. I had ridden every mile of the ride. I had kept my blood sugar in range the entire week. I had eaten more calories than I thought possible, plus I did a great job staying hydrated. I loved the strong muscles in my legs.

My next challenge started after the ride; I couldn't recover. I slept plenty. I got massages. I saw my acupuncturist. I took long, slow walks. Strangely enough, I felt more worn out, more exhausted than I had ever felt in my life. I was thirty-nine years old and I realized I was scared, but I didn't know what I was scared of.

I called Dr. Matt and told him how I felt. He agreed with me: It didn't make sense. He sent me in for a battery of blood tests. One test I had was a glycosylated hemoglobin, known as an A1c, as I've mentioned earlier. It came back 9.2%. That also didn't make sense. The numbers on my blood glucose meter didn't correspond to this high A1c. Dr. Matt had me testing almost every two hours, including all night long, to see if there was a time where my blood sugar was skyrocketing and we didn't know. My testing did not reveal such a gap, and none of the other blood tests revealed anything. This was all happening in 2004, which was before the days of continuous glucose monitors. (In someone who doesn't have diabetes, an A1c is generally below 5.7%.)

About three months after the 400-miler, I was in Detroit for work and was having a hard time falling asleep. There are acupressure points on the chest that are calming. While pressing these points, I felt a lump in my right breast. Instantaneously, the fear I had been carrying for months reared its head; I knew this was serious business. I'm not a pacer, yet that night, I paced back and forth in the hotel room. I can still see the room's cream-colored walls, multicolored bedspread, and artwork on the walls. I called my friend Chris to get comfort and advice. Chris advised me to call my primary care physician the next day and make an appointment immediately. I did. The day I got back to Denver, I went in to see her. On October 20, I got the news: I had breast cancer.

SURVIVING CANCER TREATMENTS

Thus began the endurance sport of surviving breast cancer treatments.

The first challenge was to find an oncologist I liked and trusted. Luckily, a high school friend, Lia Gore, who's a pediatric oncologist, lived and worked in Denver. Her mother happened to have been my high school Spanish teacher and was a breast cancer survivor. Lia has regular checkups to make sure she doesn't have breast cancer. She knew several highly regarded oncologists who specialized in breast cancer in young women in Denver. She gave me their names and I found one that I liked.

Then began two months of constant doctor visits and tests. I had to have my entire body scanned to determine if there was cancer anywhere else. Thankfully, there wasn't. I also had to have my teeth cleaned because, once the chemotherapy started,

I could get mouth sores that might not heal for a while, so starting off with clean teeth is wise. I had my heart and lungs tested and my bones analyzed. As a person who had lived at this point for twenty-three years with type 1 diabetes, I thought I understood the medical world. Entering the cancer world is a whole other ballgame. For one, my appointments were scheduled and coordinated by office managers at the doctor's office. This was completely new and reminded me how serious cancer is.

Tears welled up on a regular basis. The dramatic nature of the attention, the focus, the need to act with speed got to me daily. I was thankful for my meditation practice as it reminded me to slow down even if just for a moment every hour. One of the scans took over an hour and the liquid they pumped into my body (to see how it reacted with fast growing cells) chilled me to the bone. While I breathed deeply and thought of warm, sandy beaches, it came to me to get new winter boots. As soon as the scan was finished, I drove to REI and picked out a stomping warm pair of Sorel boots that made the cold of the scan fade.

LOSING MY HAIR

I continued to work at my school coaching job through the start of chemotherapy, which began in December 2004. A few days before New Year's, I went to see my hair stylist, Maria. She cut my hair super short. Then, on New Year's Eve, my sister shaved my head because my hair was falling out in clumps. Many people sent beautiful hats and scarves, so I had head covering options. I discovered I had a well-shaped head, not something those who have hair usually know about themselves. I didn't feel great being bald, but given all that I was going through, the hair loss didn't consume me. I figured it would grow back.

My sister has a minor obsession with wigs, so we went on a wig-shopping extravaganza. We found a "red long hair with bangs" wig that I wore a grand total of five times when I was completely bald. When my cancer journey was over, I gave the wig to my sister, who has been known to have parties where everyone wears a wig.

My work at the time was coaching Big Picture Learning high school teachers and school leaders in how to do project-based learning and experiential internships in their schools. These were all around the country, which meant flying all over the United States. I boarded the planes wearing my wig or a headscarf, hopeful that no one on the plane would wonder what was happening with me. The identity of "in cancer treatments" didn't feel good, so I attempted to hide it. Thankfully, as my hair fell out, my energy waned and I got more comfortable with the treatments; I tossed my fear of judgment to the wind. I began telling anyone who was curious that I was surviving cancer.

LEARNING TO RECEIVE

In Detroit again, the community at one of the schools pulled me into a spontaneous, beautiful prayer circle. It was at the edge of the school lounge area, light streaming in the windows. They pulled me into the center of the circle they formed around me. There were about twelve or fifteen people gathered around me, putting their hands on my head, arms, shoulders, and back. Everyone had their eyes closed. Someone started speaking in a quiet, strong voice, asking God to help heal my body.

Inviting the Holy Spirit to have mercy on me, and heal the cancer moving in my body. Others joined in, telling God that I was a good, helpful person, and I needed God's help today. To please come and hear the prayer, the call for help. Never before had I been the focus of a prayer circle. My heart was profoundly touched by this generous show of love and kindness. Slowly, I was learning how to receive. I had taken comfort most of my life in always being a giver. Cancer threw me to the ground, and I had the opportunity to learn to receive. It didn't come easily to learn how to open my heart and allow myself to simply receive in the spirit of all I had previously given.

Another surprise was that for the first four months after telling the world I had cancer, six days a week, a card or a gift arrived in the mail. Things arrived from all over the world as I knew people who lived in many places due to the work I had done at more than ten high schools, and at a leadership camp in California. Day after day, opening these cards and gifts sent with so much love and thoughtfulness, I felt my heart opening bit by bit.

CHEMO AND RADIATION

I decided before starting chemo that I would ride my bike as much as possible; I didn't want to lose all my fitness. I intuited correctly that exercise would help me make my way through treatment. Throughout chemo, I mounted my bike on the trainer in the living room, and I rode as many days as possible in fifteen-minute increments. On one wall in front of me, I had a poster of a Tour de France team. On the other wall, I had a photo of Coach Nicole and her professional cycling team. These two teams kept me going. My physicians, and

Coach Nicole, advised me not to ride my trainer longer than an hour a day. Anything longer could begin to break down my immune system, which was getting a massive cancer treatment workout. My chemo cycles lasted two weeks. Days one through four were awful. By day five I usually started to feel human and could ride again. I would ride through day 14 and then start the cycle over.

A few months after chemo ended, it was time for radiation therapy. It was newly spring, and the radiation treatment center was only four miles from my house. I biked there for as many days as I could. The staff accommodated me by letting me store my bike in an unused office for safekeeping. This was my expensive LeMond bicycle that meant the world to me; not letting it get stolen was high on my list of priorities.

I rode my bike to and from radiation eighteen times, exactly half of the sessions. Coach Nicole had races in Colorado, and she was able to ride with me to and from radiation three times. Riding my bike during chemo and radiation didn't preserve my fitness to perfection, but it gave me a sense of control over my destiny. Going through cancer treatment can feel like victimization, an antidote to which is to discover where one still has power. For me, that was exercise.

MY FIRST TRIATHLON

Toward the beginning of my thirty-six radiation treatments, I met a cancer survivor who coordinated events for other survivors in the Denver area who liked to be athletic. She invited me to come meet some of them at a Danskin Triathlon event. I was intrigued.

I showed up to the Survivors' Breakfast the Saturday morning before the triathlon and met about thirty women, all of whom were cancer survivors and all of whom planned to do the all-women sprint distance triathlon the next morning. I met Sally Edwards, the official spokesperson for the Danskin Triathlon, which later became the Trek Women's Triathlon Series. Sally was the main speaker at the morning gathering. At the time, she'd completed sixteen Ironman distance (2.4-mile swim, 112-mile bike, 26.2-mile run) triathlons and authored the first book about triathlons. Sitting on the edge of the picnic bench, one week away from having finished thirty-six radiation treatments, I was now on short-term disability due to a concentration disorder from the chemo and radiation. I made the decision to do the full sprint distance triathlon the next day. That's how inspired I was hearing Sally speak. Sitting among these cancer-surviving women, I knew I wanted to do this new athletic event.

The chemo and radiation had worn me down so badly that I was diagnosed with the concentration disorder. Meaning that I was unable to concentrate on anything longer than about five minutes. After five minutes, I would forget what was happening in a television show, or what I was listening to on the radio. This happened when I was attempting to answer emails or talk to colleagues on the phone while working. I couldn't even read books, that's how short my ability to focus and concentrate had shrunk. My doctors said things like this sometimes happened when people went through cancer treatments. My main oncologist and a social worker strongly encouraged me to stop working and let my body and mind rest. I finally agreed. The only thing I was able to do was take long walks and go on short bike rides on routes I knew, as due to my concentration challenges, it was very easy to get lost. I was ready for an exercise challenge. Triathlon here I come.

After the Survivor's Breakfast wrapped up, the first thing I did was go to the race registration tent where they were selling triathlon gear. I realized I didn't have a swimsuit anymore, but I discovered triathletes swim, bike, and run in the same outfit. I purchased my first-ever triathlon outfit. I liked it. It felt good, which was a delightful surprise. As with my discovery that wearing comfortable, tight-fitting bike clothing improved my performance on the bike, the triathlon outfit fit me well and dried off quickly. And I liked the colorful design of the outfit, always a plus. Having the gear of the event helps you fit in with the others doing the race. Even though this was my first triathlon, having the outfit boosted my confidence.

I got my race number, official swim cap, and the special Team Survivors shirt. Then I drove home and dug out an old pair of swim goggles. I ate some lunch and drove to the nearest pool. I asked the attendant how many laps equal a half-mile; he said thirty-two laps, which is sixty-four lengths. I took a deep breath and jumped into the pool.

As I very slowly swam those thirty-two laps, I realized I hadn't swum seriously since I was a freshman in high school on the swim team. I quit the swim team after three weeks because I had to do flip turns and putting my head below my heart made me dizzy: lowish blood pressure, I learned later.

The sprint distance triathlon was a half-mile swim in a reservoir followed by a 12-mile bike ride and 3-mile run. Once I successfully swam thirty-two pool laps, I knew I could finish the triathlon the next day. This was a big endeavor on many levels. My goal for this race was to simply finish. My time doing the event did not matter. I had not trained at all for any of the events of the race, other than riding my bike for short distances and going for regular walks. I had not swum and I had not run. It was the courage to simply sign up, show up, and complete the event that mattered. I figured if I had survived cancer treatments, I could survive this triathlon.

I was assured in my ability to bike 12 miles, and I figured, worst-case scenario, I could walk the 3-mile "run." With absolutely zero knowledge about triathlons, I packed my gear, cleaned my bike, and hoped I had enough gel packets; in case I ran out of energy or my blood sugar dropped, I could eat these while out on the course. Then I ate a good dinner and went to bed early, intentionally not telling a soul that I was going to do this event. I wasn't 100 percent convinced I would finish and had no idea what I was getting into. This was a risk I wanted to take by myself. Signing up to do this event reminded me of signing up to do The Bicycle Tour of Colorado. I wanted to see what I was made of. My chronic illnesses had not killed me, and I wanted to see what this body could do.

I woke up several hours before the race was to start, had breakfast, loaded my gear into the car, and drove twenty minutes to the reservoir. My first surprise of the day was the long line of cars headed to the race venue. I was forty years old and had never competed in a running race or triathlon. I had done a grand total of one big bike event: The Bicycle Tour of Colorado. I was a newbie. Back to those mantras. I had to reassure myself that I was brave, that I belonged here, that it was OK to ask a lot of questions. I kept reminding myself that I was an athlete, even if I barely had hair and I was wearing my brand-new triathlon outfit.

I found where to get my race number written in black marker on my calf, arm, and hand. Because I was a cancer survivor, I had a special place to rack my bike and set up my transition station. Since I barely knew what a transition was, I was grateful when a kind woman, herself a cancer survivor, gave me a few tips on how to set up my gear at the transition. Then, all the cancer survivors went to line up at the water's edge. I quickly realized that all the cancer survivors were in one "wave" right behind the professional athletes. Wearing pink swim caps, there were less than twenty of us and we had various levels of experience doing triathlons. In a few minutes it was clear that I was the newest to it. I kept asking lots of questions as we waited for our start. We watched the speedy pros go off and then a few minutes later it was our turn. I saw Sally as I was about to run into the water. That gave me a burst of courage. I knew I could swim as slowly as I needed to. I tuned into my body and felt my strength.

I swam slowly and steadily. Lots of people ended up passing me, and luckily in that first triathlon, no one bumped into me. Rather miraculous! I discovered again the joy and beauty of swimming in open water. It was calming. I made it out of the water and noticed that lots of the women were running from the water to the transition area. I walked slowly. I knew I needed to conserve my energy, since I still didn't have any reserve from all the cancer treatments.

I didn't know that they timed the transitions, so I took my sweet time. I tested my blood sugar, went to the porta-potty, and slowly put on my bike shoes and the Survivor singlet. I even took a moment and walked around looking at bikes in the transition area. In all, that first transition took me more than eight minutes. With my experience now, it was an age.

The bike ride was lovely. It felt good to be on my bike riding near other people with the same goal—to enjoy and finish. I ate a gel packet and drank some nutrition in my water bottle. Thankfully my blood sugars didn't go up or down and stayed steady. I smiled that entire ride. I felt whole and part of something bigger than me, my cancer, my trauma, and my diabetes. I experienced wave after wave of belonging. I said hello to everyone who wasn't racing like the devil was chasing them, which was quite a few people. Pure enjoyment down to my toes.

I made it off the bike with grace and ease. I re-racked my bike, took off my bike shoes, and put on my run shoes. At this point in my life, I was in no way a runner, so my run shoes at this point were a pair of old sneakers I used for taking long walks. They didn't fit the way you want and hope run shoes will fit, and they were rather worn out, but what did I know at this first triathlon? A grand total of nothing!

I had found an old fanny pack and stuffed into it my blood glucose testing device, a bunch of glucose tablets, and a few gels. I put that on and went over to the run start. Moved by the enthusiasm of the spectators who cheered for me because of my singlet "TEAM SURVIVOR," which declared that I was a cancer survivor, I began the run by attempting to run.

That lasted for about 100 yards. I quickly ran out of running juice. At this point in my life, I had trained for exactly zero running events. I was a fast walker, so I walked as fast as I could for the majority of the 5K. A few times, my enthusiasm bolstered me and I jogged a few yards.

I used the walking and sometimes running time to think about what a good experience I was having. I breathed deeply and kept realizing over and over how part of it I felt. How I had found a place I belonged. I enjoyed being celebrated for surviving cancer treatments. I enjoyed being part of a group of people swimming, biking, and running together. I found myself wondering if there were more of these triathlons. Could I repeat this joy over and over again?

I wondered if I could find a triathlon coach and train for all three of the events, not just the cycling. I knew from my biking experience with The Bicycle Tour of Colorado that time and training make all the difference.

Coming up toward the finish line, many spectators of the women doing the race had gathered with cowbells and signs to cheer on their athletes. Because of my singlet, I stood out too. People cheered me on. Their love and enthusiasm propelled me to pick up my pace and run a bit more than walk. It caused tears of joy and accomplishment to start leaking out of both eyes. Crossing the finish line was one of the most powerful celebrations of accomplishment of my life. I knew that things were changing for the better in my life. Remember, you too can cross a finish line. Best thing, you don't need to get cancer to make it happen.

THE POWER OF SETTING GOALS AND SIGNING UP

My whole life I've liked setting goals. I discovered leadership in second grade when I organized a penny drive for children who had less than those of us at our school. I realized that I needed to know how much I wanted to raise in order to tell prospective donors why they should give to the cause. I needed to know how many classmates I had to recruit so that we could reach the goal. To arrive at a desired outcome, I wanted to first visualize it, the end result, the goal.

Turns out this is a valuable way of thinking and acting in endurance athletics. What's the first athletic goal that comes to your mind? Maybe it's a 5K run or 60-mile bike ride or sprint distance triathlon. Could be it's a bigger goal, a BHAG: an Ironman, a marathon, a 100-mile bike ride. Write it down today. Writing things down helps make them real.

Now, imagine doing it. Visualize *all* of it. See yourself in your race garb. Picture yourself owning the required gear. Hear people cheering for you. Feel your health, or weight, or the wisdom that comes with age, working to your advantage. Allow yourself to feel and know all your gifts and talents working for you at this moment.

Mentally stand at the start line. Allow both your excitement and nerves to exist. Hum the national anthem. Notice your fellow participants preparing to do the same event you will do. See yourself starting. See your body moving powerfully during each part of the event.

See the finish line in the distance. Near it, and then successfully cross the line. You did it! Soak in the emotions of accomplishing your goal. Even now, in this moment of imagining it all. This will help you make it real.

POWER OF VISUALIZATION

The power of visualization is a big deal. Take Olympic athletes. It turns out that the athletes who picture themselves crossing the finish line first are more likely to do it. According to Ellen Rogin and Lisa Kueng, authors of *Picture Your Prosperity: Smart Money Moves to Turn Your Vision into Reality*, it's not just physical training that leads to success.

What makes visualization such a powerful technique for success?

Rogin and Kueng describe it as conditioning for your brain, suggesting that you first establish a goal, visualize achieving that goal in detail, and focus on it over the long term.[3]

I know from repeated personal experience how visualization has made a positive difference in my life. This book you are holding in your hands? Done. I kept visualizing you holding it as I was writing and revising it. To celebrate being finished with this book, I trained for my second ever full marathon running race. I visualized what I would wear, and how I would train my body to be able to run all 26.2 miles.

THE BELIEVING GAME

It's time to create a plan to be able to make your athletic goal a reality. Take a deep breath and remind yourself that you are smart and resourceful. The universe will support you in accomplishing this goal. You might not 100 percent believe it just yet, so play what Peter Elbow[4] dubs "The Believing Game." (A game in which you decide to believe everything that you want to accomplish *is* possible.) You act *as if* it is possible and doable. When you play The Believing Game, it is important to play 100 percent.

I've taught The Believing Game to many aspiring endurance athletes. I've also taught the Believing Game to high school and college students as they are working to navigate their lives. I also make a point of playing the Believing Game with myself. It works. Now it's your turn to play. The key is to simply let your doubts wash away, and to believe that you can do what you imagine yourself doing.

PICK A SPECIFIC EVENT

Imagine the sport and distance in which you will participate. Now find an actual event that matches your ambitions. Ideally, it's far enough in the future that you'll have time to train for it.

How to find events? Hop online and Google events that are geographically close to you. For example, a few years ago I Googled "100-mile bike rides in the Twin Cities" and all kinds came up. One of my favorite websites for finding events is www.active.com, which lists events in all kinds of categories such as triathlons, bike events, and running events.

After I did that first Danskin triathlon, I was so happy crossing the finish line to all that cheering. People didn't know who I was, but because I had on a shirt that said "TEAM SURVIVOR," everyone knew that I was a cancer survivor, and they cheered and clapped extra loud when they saw me. I walked around after the race soaking up all the love and community.

At the Danskin triathlon I saw a booth for the Denver triathlon club "Team CWW," for Colorado Wild Women. I'd had such a good time doing the triathlon that I gathered all the information and, after a bit of research, decided I would join the club the following year.

That next year, more than three hundred women showed up to Team CWW's kickoff event. I was blown away. I had no idea that many women wanted to do triathlons. A few weeks later, Team CWW had small gatherings all over the Denver area. The idea being to connect women who lived near one another so that we could go out on runs, bike rides, and swims together. I attended one in my neighborhood, sitting and talking with women who ended up becoming dear friends for years because we swam, biked, and ran together for months on end. This is the power of noticing what's happening around you at events you participate in. You will meet people who share your passion for health and wellness.

Team CWW had a number of outstanding coaches who coordinated training sessions in all three sports. The head coach was Yoli Casas, who helped me prepare for my half Ironman (1.2-mile swim, 56-mile bike, and 13.1-mile run) and later for a full marathon. Yoli, along with Nicole Freedman, were my first introduction to the power and wisdom of finding coaches to help on the athletic journey. More on the value of coaches coming up in the next chapter.

Take another deep breath. Have you found your event you will sign up for yet? Have you paid money for the event? Signing up and paying money makes your athletic goal real. I believe in you. You can do it.

TRY THIS

Journal

Step 1: Write down the name of the event/race you want and intend to do. Write down the name of the event, the date of the event, the time the event will start, what the distance of the event is. Figure out how many weeks you have to train for the event/race.

Step 2: Set the timer on your smartphone for five minutes. Let yourself imagine your race. Yes, I just gave you permission to do what used to be called daydreaming. Imagine every aspect of the event. All your emotions, what you are wearing, what the start line looks like, imagine your finishing time and what the finish line will look like, what you will drink and eat as you do the event. Let your imagination go a bit wild with imagining.

Step 3: When the timer goes off, take a moment and let the visualization settle in your body. Pick up your pen and jot down a few things that stick with you. Remind yourself to play the Believing Game. Let it all be true. Set aside your doubts and the doubts the world puts on you.

Step 4: Take a moment and write down a few mantras that you can use at your event. Then start to practice saying them to yourself. Feel free to write down at least five possible mantras, more if you're so moved.

Action

Sign up for the event. Pay your money. Make it real!

Notes

1.   See Dr. Matthew Corcoran at https://www.diabetestrainingcamp.com.
2.   "BHAG," Jim Collins, https://www.jimcollins.com/concepts/bhag. html.
3.   See Ellen Rogin and Lisa Kueng at https://www.pictureyour prosperity.com.
4.   Peter Elbow, "The Believing Game--Methodological Believing" (2008). *The Journal of the Assembly for Expanded Perspectives on Learning.* 5. Retrieved from https://scholarworks.umass.edu/eng _faculty_pubs/5.

Resources

Sally Edwards https://www.heartzones.com

Book by Sally Edwards, *Triathlons for Women: Training Plans, Equipment Advice, How-to Info*

Yoli Training Team: http://yolistrainingteam.com

Mirna Valerio: https://themirnavator.com

Run Minnesota https://www.run-minnesota.org

Carmichael Training Systems: http://trainright.com

Hal Higdon running programs: http://halhigdon.com

Jeff Galloway, Run Walk Run: http://www.jeffgalloway.com/training/run-walk

Mantras for Athletes https://www.swimbikerunfun.net/posts/best-50-running%2C-cycling-%26-triathlon-mantra%27s-for-endurance-athletes

Jeff Galloway, *Marathon, You Can Do It*

Beginner Triathlon: http://beginnertriathlete.com/Membership/Comparison

Active.com https://www.active.com

Training Peaks: https://www.trainingpeaks.com

Diana Nyad, *Find A Way*

CHAPTER 6

GATHER YOUR TEAM

"Alone we can do so little;
together we can do so much."

—*HELEN KELLER*

YOU MATTER. IT ALL BEGINS WITH YOU. YOU ARE AN ATHLETE who has signed up for a race or athletic event. You are the one who will perform at your event. Maybe you are like me and focusing on yourself isn't easy to do. I had to unlearn putting everyone before me when I became an athlete. Being female in our culture often means putting others before yourself.

When I was the activities director at Harbor High School in Santa Cruz, California, I often worked sixty-hour weeks. In addition to the Spanish classes I taught, I ran the leadership/ student government program and the Link Crew (a freshman orientation and support program), along with a few support groups and a club called Friday Night Live (which helped high school students stay sober and drug-free on the weekends). I was passionate about helping students have meaningful high school experiences, and I knew that the academic classes they took only met some of their interests and needs for making high school a valuable experience. I prioritized showing up for as many activities and events as possible. Dances, rehearsals for school-wide assemblies, overnight planning and training retreats—I did it all, with love and enthusiasm. What I didn't pay attention to was my own well-being. I was last on my list of things to tend.

When I turned thirty, I started to get sick. Not normal cold and flu sick but worn-out sickness. I finally went to see a doctor, and it turned out I was on the edge of a kidney infection. Thankfully it hadn't turned into a full-blown kidney infection, but it was a symptom of not slowing down and taking care of myself. Since functioning kidneys are essential for successful diabetes management, it acted as a wake-up call. I took some time off from work, and I slept in. I thought about how I could take better care of myself. I wondered if I could unlearn putting my own well-being last.

LEARNING TO UNLEARN

Unlearning is not an easy thing to do. In fact, the unlearning I've had to do involved reciting mantras the instant I noticed myself slipping into paying attention to others and ignoring my own needs, often to the harm of my own well-being. It took me a while to learn to notice when I was slipping; since caring for others over myself was so ingrained, I often didn't realize I was doing it. Thankfully, I became better at noticing when it happened. Then it was easier to catch myself and shift my thinking to affirmations of self-care and self-focus.

Early on I was concerned that self-care and self-focus would make me a selfish, egotistical person. As far as I could tell, no one in my childhood took care of themselves first, so I didn't have role models that prioritized self-care. No one in my early life ever talked with me about the value of taking good care of myself. No surprise that I didn't understand how critical it was to tend to my own well-being. Thankfully, with wise teachers, therapists, and a few smart friends, I learned over time that prioritizing self-care didn't make me selfish or egotistical.

In fact, the more I took care of myself, the more I had to give others. That was a huge surprise. I realized that when I ate well, got good exercise, and got enough sleep, my energy was lighter, and my attitude was brighter. There's more space within me to be generous and kind. The concept of "inner space" was also a new one. It turns out that when I have health and wellness in my body (and I have self-awareness of my health and wellness), that creates a sense of space inside my mind and being. I can witness myself. Having some empty space within myself allows me to hold space for others. When I have that extra space within myself, I notice kindness and generosity open up with ease inside myself, and that comes out in genuine service for others.

CREATOR OR VICTIM

As I began to shift my awareness to self-care, I realized I needed to shift my thinking from victim to creator. Creators view the world as if they are the captains of their ships. They see room to improve and do things better. Best of all, creators seek opportunities to change their behavior. Those who assume a victim stance focus on weaknesses and they use the language of self-defeat. They put the onus on others and view circumstances as out of their control. In other words, they tend to stay stuck in patterns of helplessness. They are often unable to take responsibility for their lives and circumstances. I had a tendency, especially in moments of overwhelm, to view my circumstances as a victim. I was a victim of diabetes, or having too much work to do, and so on. Thankfully, when I got that almost kidney infection, it was an opportunity to examine my thinking and approach.

If you lean toward a victim's way of being, find a good counselor and get help examining why you are in this mode. That's what I've done a few times in my life. Remember, the victim's way of being is not your fault. Negative bias is a common response to early trauma. I understand that when I get overwhelmed and slip into victim mode, its old patterns rearing their head. I work to get support to let these unhelpful ways go.

In many ways, it is the luck of the draw that I have creator leanings. Despite that creator leaning, I have needed and benefited greatly from having excellent counselors help me sort out the many challenges I've faced. In fact, as of this book, I haven't done a triathlon longer than a sprint distance since I did the Half Ironman in 2009. It's on my "Want to Do Again" list to do an Olympic distance and even another Half Ironman before I hit age sixty-five. There are times when I get overwhelmed and sad about the wrinkles gathering on my face, and the way aches and pains don't heal up as fast as they did when I was younger. I feel like a victim of diabetes and cancer, and I want to give up and not athletically push myself anymore.

Periodically I talk about and feel the grief of decades of diabetes and three rounds of cancer with my therapist. Feeling the sadness and overwhelm in the company of the witness of my kind and compassionate therapist helps me hold the pain and loss with self-compassion. The holding allows me to once again shift into the creator space of being the captain of my ship. In this case, my athletic ship. It's not that I ignore the pain and grief, rather it's that I feel it, witness it, and even embrace it. This allows the difficult emotions to pass through me, creating within me the space needed to get back to the habits and commitment I have to my athletic self.

You too deserve to have support as you navigate your way from victim to creator. It's worth taking a bit of time to learn when you slip from creator to victim so you can move back to being the captain of your ship.

CREATOR ATHLETE OR VICTIM ATHLETE

Being a creator or victim matters when you're an endurance athlete because, as you get deeper into your training and executing your race/event, many challenges and obstacles will emerge that you will need to figure out. It gets hard. You hurt. The weather sucks. You're tired. Having a creator mindset will give you more tools to tackle and even embrace these challenges.

The bottom line is *you* are the captain of your athlete ship. Like me, you need a crew.

CEO OF YOUR TEAM

I realized that good self-care doesn't mean doing everything on my own. In fact, self-care means gathering a team around me that believes in me and that can support my athletic and wellness efforts. This is the same for you. Along the way, I learned that interviewing doctors, therapists, physical therapists, massage therapists, and acupuncturists is not only allowed but also puts me in charge of my team.

This is true for you too. You are the CEO of your team. Good CEOs interview the new members of the team and not everyone gets hired. I discovered it's advisable to ask for references and referrals if I get stuck in the hiring process. Figuring out who you want on your team is an important task because they will all work to help you achieve your athletic goals.

Recently I had my annual oncology appointment. After all, once you've had cancer, they want you to come see a medical expert at least once a year to check in and make sure everything is humming along as it should. It had been more than twelve years since my mastectomy, and a few weeks before the oncology visit, I noticed a sharp pain in my hand and arm that felt related to my shoulder and chest. It was on the right side of my body, which is the side of the mastectomy.

My current oncologist referred me to a lymphedema physical therapist named Julie. I had to do some health insurance gymnastics to get approval, but I got in to see Julie, and I knew instantly that Julie was a welcome addition to my team. It was worth the health insurance maneuvering to hire Julie. Julie is herself a triathlete and runner. She was navigating an injury, so she was extra supportive of the pain in my arm and shoulder. Over a few months, we worked together to figure out what was going on. Turns out it was mostly related to all the computer work I do, along with sitting with my chin too far up in the air as I type. I've incorporated hourly neck stretching and I bought a gua sha tool on Amazon that I use every few hours. Thankfully, all the pain in my arm is gone. Creative teammates make all the difference.

When I had the mastectomy, I chose to not have reconstruction because that side of my chest had been radiated during my first round of breast cancer. Radiated skin and tissue never fully recovers. The radiated skin was and would continue to be very thin, meaning that to make the reconstruction work, they would have to fortify the skin by taking skin from my butt or stomach. Considering I use my abs and butt for the sports I like to do, that seemed like a bad idea to me. Additionally, to have reconstruction would have meant at least an eight-hour surgery. Given how challenging it is for most anesthesiologists to manage type 1 diabetes during a shorter surgery, asking for excellent blood sugar management for an eight-hour surgery felt practically impossible.

When I had my right breast amputated on August 20, 2010, I met with the surgeon in advance and I got permission for a diabetes educator and registered nurse, Stacey Seggleke, to manage my insulin pump and my continuous glucose monitor, which gave Stacey updates on my blood sugar for the entire two-hour surgery. As a result, my blood sugar stayed in a very normal range despite the stress on my body. I asked the surgeon and the surgical team to talk about their most joyful vacations, travels, and enjoyments in life while they did the surgery. In other words, I asked them to talk about happy, upbeat topics and to avoid politics, religion, or other loaded topics. I also asked them to periodically talk directly to my unconscious self, and tell me how well I was doing and how easily I was going to heal from this procedure. When I asked the surgeon to have these sorts of conversations during the breast amputation, at first she laughed, thinking I was teasing. I most certainly wasn't. Then she thought about it and said, "Yes, we can for sure do that. In fact, I like this idea. I will prepare a few questions to ask the team on these topics. Great idea!"

The surgery went well. In my mind it made a difference that the surgery team had upbeat, affirming conversations with one another, and directly to me while I was unconscious. I think it also made it easier on my body to navigate the trauma by having my blood sugars so closely monitored by Stacey the nurse, which resulted in keeping my blood sugars in a close to normal range, instead of ending the surgery with blood sugars in the super high range, which often happens.

I had ordered myself a Hawaiian print hospital gown and asked hundreds of friends, colleagues, and extended family to wear Hawaiian shirts on the day of my surgery, and to send me healing vibes from wherever they were on the planet that day. Hawaiian shirts remind me of the warmth, light, and love that is available to all of us. The last helpful thing I arranged were quick before-surgery and after-surgery acupuncture treatments, both of which were administered right in my hospital bed. The hospital in Colorado (where I had the mastectomy) had and still has an integrated medicine collaboration and they have acupuncturists on staff that do short acupuncture sessions before and after surgery. Both of these sessions reminded my physical body to relax, and to remember its own healing wisdom.

Finding a surgeon and a surgery team that included acupuncturists and diabetes experts is an example of finding a team that is 100 percent present for you, the athlete. It took clarity on my part to have the audacity to ask for all that I asked from them. It also required that I have confidence that what I was asking for would help my physical and emotional being recover well, which is what I was clear that I needed and wanted. It meant that I was the CEO of my body, mind, and spirit. You too can do this as you consider who you want on your team.

FIRE WHEN NECESSARY

Being the CEO of your own body, sometimes you need to make the hard call when something or someone isn't working to your benefit. Along those lines, I've had to fire a team member when their interest dropped off or they were clearly no longer looking out for my best interests or even their own. After all, I want them to be outstanding role models, so I want my team members to take good care of themselves, as well as look out for me, and my athletic efforts.

In addition to firing that early unhelpful endocrinologist (who offered no assistance, only critiques, and shamed my failure to manage my diabetes with perfection), in recent years I've had to fire an orthopedic surgeon. I went to see this doctor after I fractured a rib when I fell hard on it in the process of falling off the toilet (due to being very dizzy and nauseous as a result of a negative reaction to some of the colonoscopy prep drugs that I had been given).

The fall was intentional, because I was afraid if I didn't intentionally get from the toilet to the floor, I might lose consciousness and severely hurt myself, so I purposefully relaxed into a fall from the toilet to the bathroom floor. The fall caused my elbow to jam into my rib and the force of the fall downward onto my elbow resulted in a small rib fracture. Thankfully, it was mild enough that I could still proceed with the colonoscopy later that day. But the rib was slow to heal and when I finally went in to have it checked out, it was fractured and the orthopedic surgeon I saw was dismissive and directive about instructions that clearly had nothing to do with who I am and how I take care of myself. He knew next to nothing about nutrition and he didn't make any effort to get to know me. Instead, he told me I needed to immediately start drinking several glasses of dairy milk every day, to increase my calcium intake. He said if I didn't do that, I would hit age seventy-five and have a body full of brittle bones that would break every other minute. Needless to say, my first action was to fire that orthopedist. I will not be consulting with him on my bone health ever again. He didn't bother to ask me about my twice weekly weightlifting, my three times a week running practice, or the calcium supplements I was taking.

I want and need members of my team to be aware of nutrition and to be interested in the preventative, wellness efforts I make every day. I am open to suggestions. In fact, I love learning and making wise adaptations to my routines. My requirement is that these suggestions come from people who are in tune with science and who are willing to tune into who I am and what I am already doing. You too deserve a team who takes you seriously and who values your goals and aspirations. You are worth it! Make the effort to find the right people for you, it will make all the difference.

YOU DESERVE SUPPORT

Support is an essential part of being human. All of us are hard-wired for connection. We are social and interdependent beings. This isn't always easy for me to remember, having had a challenging childhood, and spending quite a bit of time alone as a child. One of my earliest memories is of being alone in my bedroom in a crib by myself. I didn't think anyone actually cared if

I existed. I believed this deep in my being, well into adulthood. In fact, it wasn't until the excellent therapy I got after my suicide attempt in 2013 that I unpacked this subconscious belief that no one cared if I existed. I was surprised to discover that I had friends and acquaintances that noticed my suicide attempt and cared about my well-being.

In some regards, I consider myself lucky that I have found amazing psychotherapists that have helped me examine the difficult experiences and beliefs I developed growing up in my childhood household. As I mentioned, I interview therapists before engaging long term with them. I've also learned how to ask friends and trusted medical people for recommendations. I am also good at Googling and finding Yelp-type reviews of therapists. I like therapists who understand the mind-body connection, who have done a good variety of training to get where they are, and who continue to attend training to develop their skills. I ask them questions about their education and ongoing training when I do my intake interviews. After all, these are people you want to trust so that you can let down your guard and examine vulnerable, hurt places within yourself.

Early on, I believed I only mattered if I contributed and accomplished, which is a lot of pressure to constantly perform. Because of the years of excellent therapy I've done, I've slowly and surely reframed my childhood and my early aloneness, and relearned that because I exist, I matter. My accomplishments and contributions are wonderful, but they are not what make me valuable. This has been a slow one to incorporate into my daily life. I often still benefit from reminding myself that I have a wide circle of people whom I love and who love and value me for me, not for my résumé.

Learning this did not happen overnight. In the lonely moments, I remain grateful to my dogs, who are not only terrific at getting me out of the house to walk and run, they also remind me that I'm valuable just for existing. On my journey toward becoming an endurance athlete, the friendships I've made and the coaches I found made it all possible. I believe the adage "You are who you surround yourself with."

You know your challenge. You have your event selected. You have a training plan. Now it is time to gather the members of your team.

MEMBERS OF TEAM YOU

Member #1: You

Name yourself the captain. You are the leader of your team. This may seem obvious, and I learned as a classroom teacher and later a facilitator, it's critical to state the obvious. It's a reminder to yourself and to anyone listening to you. Take a deep breath and feel and announce to yourself, "I am the leader of *my* team."

Member #2: Your physical and mental healthcare professionals

I include my endocrinologist, oncologist, acupuncturist, and psychological therapist in this section of my team. As needed, I add my massage therapist, physical therapist, registered dietitian, certified diabetes educator, chiropractor, and various sports medicine doctors I hire. I can trust all of them to help me pace myself and keep my attention on my physical and mental wellness. Who are your people?

Member #3: Coaches

You can function for a while without a coach, but I don't advise this for the long haul. Coaches are essential for your athletic improvement. I know having coaches along my journey has been a powerful addition.

Most recently, I've become a stronger, more focused runner, largely due to the influence of my coach. That's because he helps me concentrate on things I wouldn't have thought of on my own. My triathlon friend Jenny convinced me to join Run Minnesota, which offers half-marathon and marathon training programs in the spring and fall seasons. I joined and got so motivated I became a team leader for the 12-minute mile pace group. Having Head Coach Danny Docherty, who writes the training plans and is at nearly every session to guide all of us runners, has helped me improve. Danny is humble, quiet, super-focused, and very attuned to what makes an excellent training program and what helps a runner get stronger and faster. His twice weekly emails inspire and teach small, critical details in how to move my body with ease and more power.

Seeing Danny before and at the end of most of our long Saturday runs helps me gain confidence in what I am capable of doing in terms of running. Danny himself is a really fast runner, meaning he recently ran a full marathon in 2 hours 17 minutes and 5 seconds, which was a fast enough race to qualify him for the US Olympic trials. Danny understands running inside and out, and he enjoys sharing his knowledge with people like me who don't know that much about how to become a better, faster, stronger runner.

Find an Excellent Coach

Free training plans abound on the Internet. If that's the avenue you want to go down, I list training resources in chapter 11. After my one-year recovery from plantar fasciitis, I started running again and used a free app on my smartphone called Couch to 5K, which helped me gain confidence in running again.

Nonetheless, it is absolutely worth the time and money to find a coach you respect and admire, no matter where you are as an athlete. Working with Coach Yoli Casas in Colorado as I improved my triathlon skills and trained for my first marathon, and working with Coach Nicole Freedman as I became a better cyclist, made a huge difference in my progress as an athlete. Coaches learn who you are, what your goals are, and they use their experience and wisdom to give advice and guidance. It's worth it to make the investment. To help you out, here are my top seven reasons to get a coach.

Seven Reasons to Get a Coach

1. Role model expert—A good coach is accomplished in the sport they are coaching you. Here I am stating the obvious, but if you're like me searching for my first coaches, I didn't know how important it is to find coaches who really are good at the sport they are coaching. When I found cycling coach Nicole Freedman, it impressed and reassured me that Nicole had been a professional cyclist for many years, winning several national titles and competing in the Olympics. In short, she knew what she was doing. (For some extra humor, Nicole is short!) Yoli Casas, my first marathon and triathlon coach, has advanced degrees in exercise physiology and applied kinesiology, and she has competed in more than ten international marathons and scores of swimming events and triathlons. My coaches are smart and reliable: experts in what I wanted to learn. That continues to be true.

2. Accountability—Having a coach holds your feet to the fire. While I consider myself disciplined, I get sidetracked and distracted. Knowing my coach checks on me and my workouts (especially when I was training for the Half Ironman and had nine workouts a week) got me out the door and doing what was on my training plan.

3. Motivation—A coach helps motivate you when you stop believing in yourself. There are all kinds of different coaching relationships. My favorite is when the coach knows my goal and designs my training plan with me in mind, and then we have regular check-ins. When I started to doubt myself, which happened often in the early years of my athletic career, my coaches reminded me that I was capable and could do it. They reminded me of specific successes I'd accomplished, and why it was worth it to keep going.

4. Another set of eyes—It's possible to get so caught up in training that you lose perspective. Having a coach as a sounding board is ideal. For those of us with a challenging health condition or history, it's easy to get discouraged when, say, you just don't have the energy to train. Having a coach to talk to helps immensely. Nicole is the one who taught me about measuring stress in my life. Keep reading this chapter for information on the Stress Score system.

5. Focus—As a result of being an athlete, I learned a new, deep level of how to focus. Before endurance athletics, I thought I understood focus. Turns out I didn't. When I first started training, I used exercise sessions as time to mentally process the work and life challenges I was having. The more athletic I got, I realized that was a disservice to my athletic self. Slowly and surely, I learned to use the sessions as meditation, to allow my thoughts to come and go and to not get attached to the thoughts. Instead I paid attention to what was happening in my body. I discovered that my body was fascinating and subtle. There was so much to pay attention to. This deepened my body awareness and transferred to my overall wellness, because I now notice if my immune system is getting weak. I also notice subtle changes in my diabetes management. Once I got good at allowing that, I noticed an improved level of performance. Having a coach reminds me that I am worth focusing on what is happening in my body as I'm training. The coach gets me to tune in.

6. Resources—To this day, the bike-handling skills Nicole taught me informs my cycling. When I bike commute to work, at times I will ride no-handed, something I learned from Nicole. Being able to handle my bike with ease helps keep me safe on the road. Riding no-handed reminds me that most of bike control comes from my core and legs, not from my hands and arms. Nicole also taught me what to wear when it's cold outside. For her part, Yoli introduced the idea of choosing to have fun the whole race and how to tackle my fear of open-water swimming. Professional athletic coaches are networked and keep up with the latest in their sport, information that they share with you.

7. Celebration—You will reach milestones as you proceed in your training, and sometimes friends and family won't get it. Your coach will. It's important to celebrate your accomplishments, and a good coach will be there for you, singing your praises and reminding you how awesome you are!

How to Find a Coach

As for where to find a coach, if you live in a city, chances are good you can find someone locally in the race/event you want to do. It's like finding a doctor you like and respect. Ask around. Use Google. Read reviews. Meet the person in-person or over Zoom and ask lots of questions. It's an interview; after all, you will hire this person for a period of time. Hiring someone online is another way. See the end of this chapter for resources for finding an online coach.

Member #4: Friends/family who support you

As mentioned, we are who we surround ourselves with. Which of your friends and family believe in you and support your athletic goals? Not all of your friends or family will be able to relate. Identify them, too, and limit (with these people) conversations about your athletic plans. Conserve your energy and spend more of your time and enthusiasm with those who can and do support you.

Member #5: Friends/family who will train with you

In the event that your close family and/or friends do support your athletic endeavors, maybe one or two of them are willing to become athletes with you. Recruit them to join you. Having a consistent exercise buddy will go far.

Be sure to pay attention to their athletic skill level. When I was in contact with my brother and sister on a regular basis, and I was getting started with my athletic journey, it quickly became obvious that it was fun to sign up together for a marathon or a triathlon and compete on the same day. However, training together was out of the question because both were much faster than I was. Their speed had the impact of discouraging me rather than motivating me. I found friends that were closer to my speed, and together we worked on improving our times. There are days when I don't want to train and knowing I have a good accountability system reminds me to make the effort to stick to my training plan and do the workout sessions.

Member #6: Club or group you can join

I loved the years I was a member of Team Colorado Wild Women, known as Team CWW. The camaraderie and laughter made the workouts and talking about the workouts and upcoming races fun and enlivening. I made lifelong friends— friends who care about their health and wellness, who every year find fun races and adventures, who share their successes and discoveries. And, yes, friends who can be vulnerable about their occasional failure to accomplish a goal they set for themselves.

When I moved to Minnesota, it took me a while to find a triathlon team to join. The team I joined is informal, in that none of us are athletic coaches, and triathlon is more of a way to stay fit and healthy and have fun, rather than a hardcore competition. What I like best about the group is that we hold each other accountable, we work to stretch each other to do more and try harder, and we laugh quite a bit at every workout.

Ways to Find a Training Group

Google is your friend in finding training groups. Here are a few of my favorites:

- www.trifind.com lists triathlon clubs and coaches in nearly every state.
- www.meetup.com has all kinds of running, cycling, cross-country skiing, and triathlon clubs in nearly every state. Many have no membership fees.
- usacycling.org/clubs
- Many local bike shops offer group rides.
- www.runnersworld.com/for-beginners-only/how-to-find-your-ideal-running-group: This is a great article for how to find a running group that's perfect for you.
- Look into your local gym. Many gyms have started to have endurance coaches on staff and offer training programs for specific endurance events, often in running, cycling, or triathlon.
- When you sign up for an event, see if they have a training group or program you can join to help you prepare. Many sprint distance triathlons offer this, as do a number of cycling and longish running events.
- Ask on your social media accounts if anyone knows of a group you could join. After all, as an early mentor used to say to me, "If you don't A-S-K, you don't G-E-T."

KNOW YOURSELF AND KNOW YOUR STRESS SCORE

Knowing yourself is a critical step in putting together your team. One method to begin to know yourself is the Stress Score Chart. I realized early on that bringing people along to help me required that I know a good amount about myself so that I could articulate what I needed and wanted from the people I asked to be of assistance. The Stress Score Chart is one way to take stock of yourself and how you are managing the stress in your life.

When I attended Diabetes Training Camp (organized by endocrinologist Matt Corcoran) with coaches Nicole Freedman and cycling coach Rick Crawford, Rick and Nicole introduced the Stress Score Chart. Balancing your stress with recovery is a helpful way of looking at all of life, not just endurance athletics. The Stress Score Chart is a little like balancing your bank account at the end of every month. Take a moment and do the exercise from the following pages right now, in your health journal.

DEFINING THE PARTS OF THE STRESS SCORE CHART

To get started, it's important that we all have a clear understanding of the terminology of the Stress Score Chart.

Stress

There are different types of stress. Stress in and of itself isn't bad. Take a look at the three types of stress we use in the Stress Score Chart.

Physical Stress—Perhaps your job requires lots of heavy lifting. Maybe you're a parent or grandparent who takes care of young children you need to lift all day. Physical stress could also relate to a chronic illness with which you live. I consider managing type 1 diabetes as a physical stress as I deal with it every single day, and it requires a fair amount of energy to navigate.

Emotional Stress—This has to do with the emotional pressure you are coping with, or you feel like you are coping with. When my father was in hospice, and he and his team decided it was time to let go, and he went off of insulin. During the four days it took him to die, very difficult emotions swirled inside me every time I went to his bedside. During those four days, I gave myself an emotional stress score of 5, the highest score.

Training Stress—This is directly related to your workout plan and covers getting enough sleep, following your eating plan, and getting your workouts done. What is your stress level relative to the athletic event you intend to accomplish?

Recovery

Realizing that there are many ways to recover helps me stay hopeful and even joyful. When I put out a lot of energy to achieve an athletic goal, knowing that recovery is as important as the exertion helps me put out the energy.

Rest—Do you have time to sit and read or daydream or meditate? Do you give yourself time to chill out and let the tension of life fall off your shoulders?

Sleep—Being an endurance athlete means you need to get enough sleep. Chapter 10 is all about rest and sleep. Are you getting at least eight hours a night? I struggle with insomnia and staying asleep the whole night. As a result, I regularly assess and reassess my nighttime routines. I don't have a television in my bedroom, and I make an effort to not look at my phone at least thirty minutes before I want to be asleep. This means I have a collection of paper books next to my bed. For me, reading is one of the best activities for helping me fall asleep.

Therapy—All kinds of things fall under the therapy category: massage, acupuncture, physical therapy, chiropractic care, mental health counseling, and energy healing. All of these help your body, mind, and spirit recover and heal, which is essential for powerful athletic performance.

RATE YOURSELF TODAY

Give yourself a rating for today. Use a 1–5 scale, with the 1 being low (meaning you barely have any of that item). The 5 means the item is high (you have a lot of whatever it is). There are six categories for which you are going to give yourself a score. There's a chart to fill out your score for each of the six categories described above.

Stress Score Chart

This chart is deceptively simple to fill out. When I'm training for an important event, I will fill out this Stress Score Chart every day for several months at a time. I do it at the end of the day. I add it into my settle-down-for-sleep ritual. It helps me focus on what is important as I am training to perform well at an athletic event.

Physical stress:	Rest:
Emotional stress:	Sleep:
Training stress:	Therapy:
TOTAL:	TOTAL:

You're aiming to balance out the two sides. If you have high physical, emotional, and training stress, ideally you'll also have high scores for rest, sleep, and therapy. This is the Art of Training as defined by many athletic coaches. Balancing the sides of the Stress Score Chart will help you have a way to maximize the benefits of the work you're doing as an athlete.

Good job becoming the CEO of your team! Consider this a major promotion in your wellness.

TRY THIS

Journal

I've got a few things for you to do now that you are the CEO of you and your team! Take a moment and spend some time considering who, besides you, is on your team.

Who is on your team? Pull out your journal and go through all six of the groups/people who are on your team.

Member 1—that's you. Take a moment and think about how it is to declare yourself the CEO of Team You. Are you comfortable declaring yourself the CEO of you? Why or why not? If not, what can you do to increase your comfort?

Member 2—physical and mental health team members. Write down the names of all the people who are involved in your life who can help you with your athletic goal. If you don't yet have a massage therapist or an acupuncturist, and you'd like to get one, write down the category and then imagine yourself finding such a person.

Member 3—coaches. Do you have a coach yet? Would you like to have a coach who can support you? If yes, spend a moment researching where you can find one. If you don't yet want a coach, breathe into that, and remember it's okay to coach yourself as you're starting out. As you coach yourself, let yourself ask around to see if there are coaches you could hire down the road. Remain open to the idea of one day getting a really good coach, no matter your athletic skill or your age. Remind yourself that having a good coach can really help you make athletic strides.

Member 4—friends and family that support you. Make a list of the names of the friends and family who you know support and encourage your athletic aspirations. Also make a list of those who are not very supportive. Make plans to spend more time with the supportive people.

Member 5—friends and family that you could recruit to join in your athletic goal. Take a look at the list of names in Member 4. Are there any of those people that would be easy to talk into joining you on your athletic journey? Hopefully there's at least one person who could be recruited. Take a moment and visualize asking them. While you're at it, imagine them saying yes! Set a date and time to talk with this person.

Member 6—clubs or groups you could join. You can do your athletic training and race/event by yourself or with just one or two other people. I've done that. It's just so much fun when you have a community of people alongside you. Take a moment and think about the event you'll do. Are there any groups or clubs doing similar events? Spend a bit of time thinking about who you might join.

Stress Score. Take a moment and go back to the Stress Score Chart. If you haven't yet done an analysis of your current Stress Score, do it now. Take a moment and reflect on if there is anything you can do to adjust/improve your stress score. Write down exactly what and when you will take action. Remind yourself, you are worth it.

Notes

1. Stress Score creators: Rick Crawford and Nicole Freedman. Learn more about Rick: https://en.wikipedia.org/wiki/Rick_Crawford _(cycling)

Resources

To learn about unlearning, the book *Think Again: The Power of Knowing What You Don't Know* by Adam Grant is a good place to start.

To find athletic coaches, here's another resource: https://www.trainingpeaks .com/find-a-coach/

CHAPTER 7

WHAT TO WEAR AND GEAR YOU NEED

"It's very important to have the right clothing to exercise in. If you throw on an old T-shirt or sweats, it's not inspiring for your workout."

—*CHERYL TIEGS*

WHEN THE SEASON CHANGES, I GET INSPIRED THINKING about what sport activities I will do for the coming season. As I consider what races and events I will do, I immediately start thinking about what I will wear on race day, and what I will wear for all my training sessions. One of my favorite parts of endurance athletics is the gear. I love gear shopping. This was a big surprise to myself and to people who know me well, seeing that I'm not a fan of shopping in general. When I reluctantly go clothes shopping, it's most often to consignment stores and to other recycled sources such as Goodwill and low-cost outlets. Buying new clothes feels excessive to me.

Shopping for athletic gear, on the other hand, makes my heart sing. All of it fascinates me, including the helmet, the sunglasses, the shoes, the bike computer, and the many components on the bike itself. If I could, I would wear workout clothes every day all day. In fact, during the pandemic of 2020, 2021, and 2022, I wore athletic clothing nearly every single day. In that aspect, I was in heaven.

Now that I have been an endurance athlete for two decades, I've accumulated quite a bit of gear. As the season changes, instead of going out and loading up on new gear, I inventory what I have. Since I live in Minnesota these days, the transition from my favorite season, autumn, to winter is often abrupt. Those few weeks give me time to pull out my cold weather gear and assess the condition of everything I use with frequency. I find out if things still fit, if anything is too worn out, or if anything is broken.

A big secret to successful fall and winter athletics is the gear. Which brings me back to my favorite part of endurance athletics, no matter the season. Let's dive into gear, since feeling comfortable in what you're wearing and what equipment you have will boost your confidence as you get out and move your body.

HOW TO GET STARTED WITH GEAR

Number one is to be mentally solid in your belief that you are an athlete. Once again, breathe into that, and remind yourself that athletes need quality gear. You deserve quality gear that will keep you safe, visible, warm, or cool depending on the season, and if you care, you might as well be fashionable. I like being endurance-sport fashionable, and sometimes I must rein myself in, because it's true, I can get a bit gear happy and get carried away.

One of my recent obsessions is fingerless mittens for cold weather running. I found a $40 pair of thumbless mittens that have a holder for a hand warmer. Then I found a $17 pair at Target that is like the $40 pair folded over to expose your fingertips for the moments that your hands start to heat up. The Target pair easily holds a hand warmer too. As you might have guessed, I love having both pairs so that I have variety for my winter runs. The good thing is that I can wear the various pairs of mittens for a variety of winter outdoor activities, such as walking my dog and cross country skiing. I like to double dip as much as possible with my gear; it makes it easier to justify purchasing high quality gear. As I accumulate more gear, if I can use the gear for more than one sport, it's easier to keep track of the condition of each item. The gear you purchase doesn't have to be the most expensive available. What matters is that it serves the purpose you need it for, and that it is sturdy and reliable.

As you're getting started with your athletic goal, keep the gear simple and as minimal as possible. You want to discover if you deeply enjoy the sport you are taking up, and you only need the minimum amount of gear to start. Additionally, remember that when you go to a gear store, it's the salesperson's job to upsell you as much gear as possible. You do not need everything they will try to sell you, so keep yourself focused on only the items you need to give the sport a good try.

Here are four things I keep in mind as I'm assessing what I need and where I will buy what I need.

FOUR STEPS FOR DETERMINING AND PURCHASING THE GEAR YOU NEED

Step 1: Research your sport to determine what you need.

I offer you a few ideas for the sports I participate in (running, road cycling, and swimming). If you're doing these sports, you can start with my lists. If your sport is a different one, you can look on websites and/or in magazines for your sport to determine what you need.

Running

For running, consider everything from the shoes to a way to carry a water bottle and nutrition. If you will run when it's dark, you might want a headlamp and reflector vest. The shoes are the most essential component. I strongly encourage you to go to a running-specific store. Fleet Feet is a national chain that has excellent service. They will analyze your gait and make specific suggestions for shoes for you. This can happen at many local running stores too. I had my run gait analyzed, and I am a Brooks Adrenaline wearer. This is a stability shoe. I wear down the outer edge of my heel rather quickly. Inside my shoes I wear Superfeet inserts that I purchase from REI for every other new pair of Brooks. I move the inserts to the new run shoes, since they can last double the time the shoes last. I have a tendency to get plantar fasciitis, so the shoe inserts help prevent a flare up of that. In general, I get a new pair of shoes every 300 to 400 hundred miles of running, sometimes sooner, if I've worn them out more quickly.

In recent years (since falling in love with running, which I wasn't sure would ever happen), I've learned about the value of having two different brands of run shoes and alternating between them on my runs. After another gait and foot analysis, the new run shoes I'm trying out are Asics GT-2000. The idea of having two slightly different shoes that are in the same family of shoes (in my case I need a stability shoe) is to help the body avoid injury. In the time I've had these two related, but different shoes, I've noticed I don't wear out my shoes as quickly and so far, no injuries.

As for additional gear for running, keep the season in mind and what you might need to stay warm or cool. Since I'm here in Minnesota, and I'm a year-round outside runner, I have Merino wool long underwear tops and bottoms. I wear the wool bottoms underneath water-resistant, slightly heavier run tights. The two layers on my legs have kept me warm up to −30 degrees Fahrenheit, along with a sock liner and a heavy pair of Merino wool socks. Another important winter gear item is a neck gaiter. They can be worn like a hat to cover your ears and the top of your head to keep the heat in, and should you get warm as you run (which does happen), you can move the gaiter off your head for a bit of ventilation. The key advantage of Merino wool is that as you sweat and your clothes pick up the moisture, you rarely get super cold. I've often said thank you to the Merino wool I'm wearing on cold run days. Granted, when you're done with the run, you will cool down quickly and you want to have clothes to quickly change into and/or put on over your sweaty run clothing.

Cold weather thankfully doesn't last the entire year, and quickly I find that from long sleeves, windbreakers, and run tights, I move to shorts and tank tops. My current favorite brand for shorts is Senita Athletics. I use my iPhone as a medical device, and thus I need to have it on my body as I run. Thankfully, most people like to have their phones with them as they exercise, so most exercise clothing has pockets for phones, which also work for skinny water bottles and nutrition packets such as gels. I have a Flipbelt brand waistband that I can strap on with Velcro and carry nutrition and hydration for when I go on a longer run.

One of my favorite coaches imparted the following wisdom: "Always leave base camp cold." If you are warm enough just standing there, you are overdressed. Another suggestion: dress as if it's 15 degrees warmer than it is. I hate being too cold or too warm so leaving home when I'm cold is really hard.

Recently, I have been training outside in the fall in Minnesota for the Twin Cities Marathon 10-mile race. When I signed up for this race, it was in the 70s. It was summer. As the temperature dropped and the wind picked up, I wasn't sure I was going to be able to keep training. But I remember someone telling me that the weather doesn't matter as long as you have the right gear. I now take notes on what I wore and what the temperature and wind levels were. While it's sort of a pain to have to track this information, it's proven to be quite valuable in cutting down my uncertainty about what I need to wear. I like to run in the morning, so I take a moment the night before to study the weather. Then I figure out what I'm going to wear before I go to bed. I lay out my clothing, so it's easy to get dressed and get out the door for the run. This keeps me motivated on cold, dark mornings when I often just want to stay in my warm bed.

At a local gym I found this very helpful chart that's adopted from Jeff Galloway's book *Marathon . . . You Can Do It!*[1] I added a few of my own notes and commentary to it, written in italics.

°F	°C	Clothing Recommendations
60+	15+	Tank top/singlet and shorts. *When it gets this warm, I make sure I'm drinking salt tabs and I wear a cooling scarf around my neck. When the humidity is high and the temperature is high, I additionally make sure I have water scheduled for the entire workout, including water that I can use to wet my cooling scarf too.*
50 to 59	10 to 15	T-shirt/tech shirt and shorts
40 to 49	4.4 to 10	Long-sleeved shirt or short-sleeved shirt with arm warmers and shorts or tights depending on how cold it feels. If there is wind, gloves or mittens. *I wear the kind that has fingers with a glove wind cover that is optional. I also wear a headband that covers my ears because I* hate cold ears!
30 to 39	-1 to -4.4	Long-sleeved shirt with a second shirt over it, tights and shorts, and heavier socks. *Smart Wool is a favorite brand of mine.* Mittens/gloves and a hat or headband over the ears. *I wear mittens since my fingers stay warmer. If it's super windy, I will also wear a wind jacket. I often use my cycling raincoat by Showers Pass.*

°F	°C	Clothing Recommendations
20 to 29	-6.7 to -4.4	Moisture-wicking top and thick, long-sleeved T-shirt; tights and shorts; heavier socks; mittens/gloves; and a hat that covers ears. *Again, at these lower temps, I would also wear a wind resistant top or jacket. Since I hate my face being cold, I would likely have a neck gaiter with me and tuck my face in it periodically. I also rub Vaseline on my face when it's cold and windy.*
10 to 19	-6.7 to -1.1	Moisture-wicking top and thick, long-sleeved T-shirt; tights; wind-resistant outer layer (for both top and bottom); heavier socks; thick mittens; and a thick hat over ears.
0 to 9	-6.7 to -12	Two moisture-wicking tops, thick tights, long underwear, wind-resistant outer layer (Gore-Tex or similar fabric), thick mittens (or gloves), face mask, a hat that covers ears, and Vaseline or Body Glide on exposed skin.
-1 to -15	below -12	Two moisture-wicking tops, thick tights, long underwear, wind resistant outer layer (Gore-tex or similar fabric), thick mittens (or gloves), face mask, a hat that covers ears, and Vaseline or Body Glide on exposed skin. Make sure you are keeping your feet warm. *I run outside when it's this cold. At these temps I use hand warmers and sometimes I put toe warmers in my shoes with my Merino wool socks. Warm feet are key to running success.*
-20 and below	below -18	Add layers as needed. *I have run outside when it's this cold and survived. It's a fun challenge! If you want, you can run on a treadmill or on an inside track. If outside, be ready for your face to get frost on it!*

The topic of what to wear depending on the weather is a popular one on the Internet, so search away. You will find lots of opinions.

The truth of the matter is each of us is different. The best key to success has been doing my own trial and error and taking my own notes. Just like for my diabetes management, I can take suggestions, but in the end I really do need to figure out my own best strategy.

Give yourself time to figure out what works best for you. Take notes and review your notes. You too will figure out the best gear for you based on the weather.

Road Cycling

For cycling, the most important piece of gear is the bike itself. Once you get serious about cycling (meaning you are riding a few times a week with regularity, and/or you've signed up for at least a 50-mile bike ride), then you need a bike that fits you well and will hold up on your rides. My first road bike, which I bought in the year 2000, cost $2,100. I still have that steel frame LeMond bike, and I still love it. It was worth every penny I paid for it. I have another road bike that's newer than that LeMond, and I go between those two bikes. Triathlon time trial bikes can cost anywhere from $950 to $9,000 or more.

In general, I strongly encourage you to test at least five bikes before you make a decision. Ideally, take someone with you to the bike shop, since bike shops can be intimidating, and you deserve to be treated with respect and be allowed to take a bit of time making your decision. Having someone with you bolsters your confidence and gives you someone to discuss the pros and cons of each bike you test, someone who isn't invested in you making a quick decision.

Once you get the bike, if you can, have someone work with you to make sure the bike fits you well. Seat height is critical. As is handlebar distance from the seat. How far you need to lean over to reach your handlebars also matters for long distances. Someone who knows how to fit the bike to your body can teach you quite a bit about comfort on long rides.

Once you've got the bike, you'll want to figure out bike shoes. Are you ready and willing to clip in and out? I still remember when I learned how to clip in and out. On my first ride that I was clipped in, I cruised slowly up to a stop sign and completely had zero muscle memory to remember to clip out. I had applied the brakes, so the bike came to a complete stop but my feet were clipped to the pedals so I couldn't move my feet to the ground. Needless to say, I tipped over and fell onto the street. Thankfully there were no cars around, and I didn't get hurt as I remembered to fall gently (meaning I didn't tighten up my muscles as I fell). In fact, as I hit the ground I started laughing. I had practiced clipping in and out before I rode, but the memory of how to do it wasn't in my muscles yet. Needless to say, that one fall taught my body to remember to clip out a few pedal strokes before coming to a complete stop.

Deciding to clip in and out is a big one. Many people are initially nervous about making the change from regular shoes to bike shoes. As I became a more serious cyclist, it became clear that I could bike faster and more efficiently with bike shoes that clip in. That's because I could both pull up and push down as I was pedaling. This helps on long rides because the up and down motions use slightly different leg muscles, thus helping your legs fatigue less.

I'm a road cyclist, so I wear full-body Lycra. The tight clothing has the least air resistance and the least likely chance of falling off your body and getting caught in the chain, which would really suck because anything getting caught in the chain would cause the bike to stop quickly, and you would fall off. Ouch. Additionally, official bike shorts have padding in the crotch and butt area, and that padding is very helpful for long rides. Another key item, don't wear underwear under your bike shorts. Underwear will chafe your body and that is not ideal. Good bike shorts have very few seams and thus nearly zero chafing. There are a lot of companies that use the term "biking shorts" for shorts that are tight fitting, but that don't have padding. Skip those shorts if you're becoming a serious cyclist. Cycling jerseys are also valuable because most of them have a few pockets along the low back. Those pockets provide storage for extra food, arm warmers, your phone, and even an extra water bottle if needed.

There are a few additional important gear items for cycling. These items are a helmet, gloves, sunglasses, and a tire repair kit. The helmet is crucial in that should you ever fall off your bike and hit your head, it will likely save you from a serious head injury. Most cycling events require that you wear a bike helmet. Make sure it fits you well, and that it sits on your head in such a way as to not slip around your head as you move. Getting the helmet to fit well is worth the extra minutes it takes to adjust the straps.

Since I'm a road cyclist, I always wear cycling gloves. I've had a few problems with my hands (namely multiple trigger finger surgeries) and the gloves have some padding in them, which helps protect my palms. Since I lean forward as I ride, the bit of padding in the gloves helps my hands manage the bike vibrations. Additionally, if I ever fall off the bike (which has happened a few times as noted) the gloves protect my hands from getting scraped up on the pavement.

Sunglasses are another valuable gear item I always wear when riding. I have a few pairs so that no matter the sun level, I have glasses. Being outside in the sunshine for hours at a time can be dangerous without sunglasses; you want to protect your eyes from sun damage. Sunburned eyes cause terrible headaches, which in turn will interrupt your athletic training. Additionally, sunglasses reduce the glare from vehicles, glass, and even water, which will help you make wise decisions about where you're riding.

One year, I led a weeklong cycling class for a group of high school students and one student refused to wear sunglasses as we rode. I'd offered sunglasses for those who didn't have them. At the end of day one, the student said he was sick of the mosquitos and gnats in his eyes, and he'd like to use the glasses for the next day. I agree with this student, and I always remember my glasses when going for a ride. Be sure you have a comfortable pair of sunglasses for your long bike rides.

Finally, make sure you have the skill and supplies to repair a flat tire. Should that happen on a ride, it is essential for confidence when going out for any significant time. I've taken a few "repair a flat" classes at local bike shops, and I've valued every one of them. Before every ride, I make sure I have a spare inner tube and all the necessary supplies to do a quick fix. I also buy slightly more expensive bike tires, so I rarely get flats.

One more important aspect to consider is having supplies to keep your bike clean and tuned up. I put oil on my bike shoe cleats at least once a week during the outdoor riding season. I have a good tire pump and I pump up my tires before every ride. I also lube my bike chain every few rides. Should I ever get caught in the rain or end up riding on a muddy day, I make sure to clean up my bike and the chain, since a little bit of care makes the bike last longer. I also take in my bikes almost every year for a complete tune-up at a bike shop. They examine the brakes and make sure the chain hasn't stretched out, plus they look at all the parts of the bike, making sure everything is in good working condition. This annual tune-up makes me feel confident on the bike when I'm going down hills at a good speed and turning corners. This care of the bike also contributes to making the bike last a long time. You and the bike are worth it.

As you get going with cycling, you might find you gather more gear. Have fun with it; you might as well look good and feel confident as you ride.

Swimming

Swimming is the only sport I'd ever officially done as a high school student. It's true. I was not a high school athlete by any stretch. I was on the swim team for a grand total of three weeks in ninth grade. As I mentioned earlier, I gave up because I couldn't do flip turns, and no matter how I tried to learn, all that happened was I got dizzy and disoriented.

Despite not being on the swim team for very long, I have always loved swimming itself, so when I discovered triathlon, I was delighted that the first sport was swimming. Since that discovery, I like to make sure I have access to a pool so I can do some laps at least once a week all year round.

The key items to have are a swimsuit and goggles. I have fun selecting a new suit every few years from the website SwimOutlet. They have fun patterns and good materials for suits. Plus, they offer guidance on suit sizing. Goggles are another important item. Swimming in a pool, the water has a lot of chemicals in it and keeping your eyes open to see where you're going is hard if you don't protect your eyes from the chlorine and other safety chemicals. When you transition to open water swimming, goggles, like sunglasses, protect your eyes from the sun and the glare on the water as you work to sight where you are going.

From there you can also get yourself paddles, a kickboard, and flippers for drills and building muscle. For outdoor lake or reservoir swimming in the summer, I strongly recommend you get a dry swim bag, called a swim buoy, that floats behind you as you swim. I put my insulin pump, my phone, and my keys in the dry bag. If I get tired as I'm swimming, I can grab onto the swim buoy as a flotation device as I catch my breath and remind myself that I'm a strong swimmer. The psychology of open water swimming catches nearly all of us by surprise now and then.

If you are swimming in cold reservoirs, cold lakes, or the ocean, you can consider buying yourself a wetsuit. They are a serious investment, and I advise renting one before you invest, to make sure it's something you'll use. I own three wetsuits and I've tried liking each of them. I started open water swimming when I lived in Colorado, and I swam in a reservoir that was very cold from winter snow runoff. Wetsuits, a neoprene cap, and neoprene booties were vital for early summer open water swimming. I used the cap and booties, no problem. My issue is that I have exercise-induced asthma, and being in cold water and wearing a tight neoprene wetsuit caused my chest to feel compressed, which caused major panic in my system. During one triathlon race, the panic got so bad that I managed to peel off the wetsuit in the water, mid-swim, and throw it to a race support kayaker, who grabbed it. I told him the name of my coach (who was well known in the Colorado triathlon community) and he returned the wetsuit to Yoli, who gave it back to me. So try as I might, I am not a fan of wetsuits, despite how they help the swimmer stay buoyant and warm. I make an effort to do open water swimming in warmer water these days. Nonetheless, wetsuits work for many people, and just because I don't like them doesn't mean they won't work for you. Many of my swimming friends much prefer open water swimming with their wetsuits.

Triathlon

I've gone through run, bike, and swim gear with some level of detail so far. Combine all of these and you have a triathlon. Fun how that works. The items you need specifically for triathlon are a good bag (to haul all your gear to and from the race and set up your transition area) and, of course, the triathlon outfit itself.

Because I wear a tubed insulin pump, I prefer a two-piece triathlon outfit, which allows me to clip my pump on the waist band. Many of my triathlon pals love the one-piece outfits. Whichever way you go, the key is to have something comfortable you can wear swimming, then biking, and then running. Except for a full Ironman race, you cannot get naked in the transition area, so you need to wear the same outfit for all three sports. Triathlon outfits are made out of quick drying material with a minimal amount of padding in the shorts, which means you should practice cycling in them before your event. I purchase a new triathlon outfit every few years, since they can start to wear out. SwimOutlet.com has triathlon outfit options too, as does the website Beginner Triathlete. They have a detailed section on gear reviews, which I find very helpful.

Step 2: Determine how much money you are willing to spend on gear and make a list of what you need.

Check off the items you already have and highlight the ones you still need. Now you know what you need to find. With athletic gear, the goal is to buy the best you can responsibly afford. There have been times when I've purchased up on an item when I knew I was going to use the item repeatedly. I did this with my ShowersPass raincoat. It's officially a cycling rain jacket, but I wear it on runs when it's raining. These rain jackets are expensive, and I've loved cycling and running in this jacket. Plus, it's held up over the years, remaining rain proof.

If finances are tight, start basic, and then purchase up on items later as experience tells you which items you find the most value in buying higher quality. In the three sports I outlined, I have found that purchasing up in key gear like bike shorts, sunglasses, and rain jackets has been well worth the money. But remember, as you're getting started, you don't *need* an expensive rain jacket; the most important thing is to start!

Step 3: Research where to purchase what you need.

You want gear that will endure. You're in this sport for physical and mental health and for the long haul; you don't want gear that's going to fall apart in less than one season. Take the time to research options and be resourceful. A store near my house sells and repairs gear for resale. I ended up purchasing a new-to-me pair of classic cross-country skis, boots, bindings, and poles at a fraction of the cost of new. I've skied on them for more than five years now, and they are wonderful. When the boots started to fall apart, rather than buy a new pair, I found a shoe and hockey skate repair shop, and they fixed up the boots to almost as good as new. I like REI and run-specific stores as well as smaller bike shops for purchasing gear. Find the stores in your area and look online. And remember, price doesn't always equal quality.

Step 4: Make the purchases.

This may seem obvious, but the truth is making a gear purchase is a step in acknowledging to yourself that you really are an athlete. It might not always be as easy as it was for me getting the skis at The Repair Lair, so remember to not give up hope. Be persistent. And always ask a lot of questions. Additionally, consult with your friends. Since I love gear, consider reaching out to me. I'd happily discuss gear options with you! For sure don't let the salespeople pressure you. Take the time you need and make good decisions.

Well done making your way through one of the most fun parts of being an endurance athlete: the gear! Finding, purchasing, and then wearing and using the gear for your sports takes you one step closer to becoming an official endurance athlete.

TRY THIS

Journal

Make a few lists:

1. A list of all the gear you have
2. A list of the gear you think you need
3. A list of where you can purchase the gear you need

How are you feeling about purchasing the gear you need? Take a moment and write about how it feels to take this next important step on your wellness journey.

Action

Go shopping for gear!

Notes

1. Jeff Galloway, *Marathon . . . You Can Do It!* (Bolinas: Shelter Publications, 2001), 170.

Resources

Swim and triathlon suits and gear: https://www.swimoutlet.com
Run shoes and clothing: https://www.fleetfeet.com
Cycling clothing: https://www.primalwear.com
Run shoes and bra that Mari wears: https://www.brooksrunning.com
Beginner Triathlete: https://beginnertriathlete.com

CHAPTER 8

ATHLETES EAT LIKE THIS

"One cannot think well, love well, or
sleep well if one has not dined well."

—*VIRGINIA WOOLF*

WHAT TO EAT? THOSE OF US WITH HEALTH CHALLENGES ASK
ourselves this question a lot. I've struggled with answering this
question. I had a rough childhood and, thankfully, one of the
bright spots was learning from my mother how to cook.

Starting when I was five, my mom made sure my siblings
and I were in the kitchen helping her make meals. This was
always a fun time filled with laughter and discovery. As I
got older, my mom had my sister, brother, and me plan and
cook dinners for the whole family. By age ten, I knew how
to make a pot of spaghetti and toss fresh greens for a salad.
This early cooking instruction serves me well as an adult.
Meaning, I learned early that cooking was fun and doable,
and that healthy meals didn't take a lot of effort. Granted, I
forgot these early lessons for a few years, and a second round
of cancer forced me to remember.

ENDURANCE ATHLETES NEED TO EAT

One thing I learned after reading countless sports nutrition books, websites, and articles (and after consulting with a number of registered sports dietitians) is that *what* you eat is up to *you*. If you want to eat meat and dairy, then eat that. If you want to eat processed food, do that. If you want to go Paleo, do that. If gluten doesn't work for you, don't eat gluten. It's your body, and what you put into it (once you're an adult) is up to you. That said, if you want to have top performance as an endurance athlete, you'll want to pay attention to what you eat, and how you perform in your sport depending on what you eat. You might need, and want, to make a few adjustments to your eating habits and patterns.

Early in my athletic career, the dietitian I worked with, (Marcey Robinson, MS, RD, CSSD, BE-ADM) described Ironman triathlons as being "swimming, biking, running, eating, drinking" competitions. I laughed when she first said this, and then, by trial and error, learned that she is 100 percent correct. Nutrition and hydration are critical components of endurance athletic performance.

Sports nutrition is a complicated field. There are scores of different theories out there about what, when, and how we should eat. I'm not going to tell you how you should eat. I am not a registered dietitian, and I am most certainly not your mother. I will share a few insights I've gained over the years, and about the rationale I use to eat the way I do when I'm training. I'll also give you some resources to explore.

EAT LIKE AN OLYMPIAN

Early in my years of being coached by and hanging out with pro cyclist Nicole Freedman, I was impressed with how cleanly she ate, meaning she tried not to eat food like chips, candy, or sweets. Junk food is, in essence, refined foods that are far from how nature made them. The food is processed so much that the fiber is removed, as is most of the food's nutritional value. Often, processed foods have vitamins or minerals added back in, but they have lost their natural vitamins and minerals. The food is so dramatically altered that now we know the gut biome doesn't have to do much to process the food in our bodies. Turns out this isn't very good for our health.

The food becomes junk because it doesn't provide the macronutrients our bodies need to live healthfully. When trying to perform endurance exercise, junk food will cause more setbacks than progress.

Clean eating, on the other hand, is defined as eating whole food—real food that is minimally processed or not changed at all from the way it grew. Think of a grain like quinoa—it is processed because it has to be taken from the plant it grew on. But the fiber, proteins, or the vital nutrients it grows with are not removed when it's picked. This allows our body to benefit. The food in clean eating is as close to its natural form as possible.

Nicole ate lots of fresh veggies and fruit. She ate eggs and grass-fed meat. I noticed this was true for my friend and Olympian Chris Klebl too.

I went through a phase of not cooking. Since I couldn't afford to eat out, I consumed a lot of Lean Cuisine frozen dinners. When I started paying attention to what Nicole and Chris ate, I realized that neither of them ever ate a frozen dinner, not even the "healthy" ones. Diagnosed with breast cancer for the second time, I decided (at the age of forty-five) that my ability to twice grow cancer from scratch was an opportunity for me to closely examine what I could control and couldn't control about my lifestyle.

First on my agenda was to look at my nutrition. I'd become a fan of Kris Carr[1] (author of the movie and book series *Crazy Sexy Cancer*) after my first round of cancer. Kris lives with a rare, incurable, slow-growing, stage IV cancer. She was diagnosed on Valentine's Day in 2003 when she was thirty-one years old. It was a huge wake up call for her. She traveled around the globe searching out healing practitioners, and she videotaped her interactions and discoveries. That became her movie. Kris discovered that a plant-based diet of nearly zero processed food was an important key to health. The typical American diet is full of processed food, and it's slowly and surely killing us.

I was eating a lot of processed food. All those Lean Cuisines weren't helping me. I ate a lot of meat and cheese, and I always had a gallon of milk in the fridge and ice cream in the freezer. I didn't eat very many fresh vegetables. I was surprised how poorly I ate, since I thought I ate well. I wasn't significantly overweight and exercised often. I thought I was super healthy, and here I had gotten cancer a second time. I needed to make a change.

My Journey to Healthy Eating

In addition to rereading everything Kris Carr had written, I read *The China Study* by T. Colin Campbell, PhD. Kris and T. Colin woke me up to my error of a cancer survivor eating dairy products and meat. I had been a vegetarian for nearly five years in my late twenties and had generally felt great. Action item Number 1 was to completely change my eating habits.

I opened the fridge, took out the gallon of milk, and dumped it down the sink. I took out the cheese and butter, and I tossed them in the trash. I opened the freezer and removed the frozen dinners and the ice cream—also into the trash. Then I took the trash out to the dumpster in the alley, not wanting to tempt myself to fetch any of these items out of the trash.

Walking back into the house, I recited to myself, "I now eat lots and lots of vegetables. I now eat clean. I can do this." I wasn't completely convinced I could, but I was willing to make a concerted effort to be an endurance athlete, a diabetes and cancer-surviving athlete who didn't eat meat, dairy, or gluten.

Gluten-Free: That Too?

Around the time I was diagnosed with breast cancer for the second time, my acupuncturist in Denver, Colorado, (Carol LeCroy) asked me for the umpteenth time to please consider giving up gluten. I loved bread and pasta and couldn't imagine life without gluten. I was suffering from horrendous hot flashes. I thought they were terrible because of having gone through chemotherapy. Carol suspected I had gluten intolerance. I'd recorded several days of hot flashes, and, on average, I was having more than twenty-seven full-body (complete with sweat) hot flashes in a 24-hour timeframe. It was wearing me out.

Carol convinced me to give gluten-free a try. Within two weeks, I had a miraculous shift in everything. The hot flashes stopped. I no longer had stomachaches. I felt energized. I was sleeping better. After a few months, I discovered I was no longer allergic to cats, which I had been deathly allergic to since I was eighteen. For the first time in many years, I didn't have seasonal allergies. Chances are good I have celiac disease. However, to get an official diagnosis, I would have to eat gluten again, and I was not, and am not, willing to do that.

Eat Clean

The question I faced now was how to eat clean as a gluten-free, nondairy, and nonmeat eating endurance athlete? The question baffled me. To be clear, clean eating overall does not mean one needs to avoid eating meat, or dairy, or gluten. In my particular case, it does mean all those things. Clean eating overall means paying attention to the quality of the foods you are eating and eating as little processed food as possible.

I did what I do when confronted with a big challenge: I started reading, and I sought the guidance of smart people around me. I read books by Canadian Ironman Brendan Brazier[2] (a plant-based endurance athlete who founded the Vega brand products sold in health food stores). One key thing I learned through his writing is that when the body goes meat- and dairy-free, it learns to process protein more efficiently, meaning that a nonmeat, nondairy eating person doesn't have to eat as much protein. What a great thing to learn.

I asked my oncologist who their clinic dietitian was and made an appointment to see her. Unfortunately, the dietitian specialized in helping people going through chemo figure out how to keep eating, which wasn't the guidance I was seeking. I then turned to my colleague and diabetes educator associate, Marcey Robinson, MS, RD, CSSD, BC-ADM, who has many letters after her name and is qualified to give sports nutrition advice. I set up a meeting with Marcey to talk about my desire to completely change my diet.

Marcey took it upon herself to research and discover what she could find in scientific studies about eating and cancer. She supported my decision to give up meat, dairy, and gluten. She suggested I also consider giving up alcohol. Her rationale was that the liver, which also happens to be the key organ that processes estrogen, processes alcohol. I had estrogen-receptor positive breast cancer all three times. Marcey suggested that it might be wise to greatly limit the times I distracted my liver from effectively processing estrogen, which alcohol would do. I took a deep breath and made the decision to limit my annual alcohol consumption to four glasses of wine a year. It's been more than twelve years since I made this decision, and that continues to be how much alcohol I drink each year, sometimes less.

Terms in the eating well world come and go depending on the trends of the moment. I refer to how I eat as "clean eating." For me, I consider clean eating to follow these basic principles:

- Minimal sugar.
- Minimal processed food of any kind, including processed vegan food items.
- No gluten.
- Minimal animal products. I do eat eggs a few times a month and these days I also eat a few cheese and Greek yogurt items, but not much.
- No caffeine.
- No soda of any kind.
- Minimal alcohol.
- Eat out as little as possible.
- Eat good fats such as olive oil, avocado oil, and avocados.
- Have fun cooking!

Learn to Cook Again

Marcey made a few other life-altering suggestions. One was to find and cook a new recipe at least once a month. Since I had pretty much given up cooking, this was a big step for me. Friends gave me vegan cookbooks, and I went to the library to check out a few more. I selected recipes that contained no gluten and had lots of veggies. I photocopied the recipes I liked and started a binder of my favorites. To this day, every month, I add to that binder.

Having survived a second cancer diagnosis, I eat clean most of the time. That said, when I'm training for a long endurance event—a run longer than 10 miles, a triathlon longer than sprint distance or a bike ride longer than 50 miles—I pay even closer attention to how I eat before, during, and after the event. When I eat clean, I notice after just a week how good eating healthy food causes me to feel. In my daily morning meditation, I notice that healthy food makes my muscles, joints, ligaments, and whole body feel strong and healthy. Making the effort is worth it. Over the years, I have slowly come to appreciate my weekly cooking sessions. As I cook for the week, I send healthy, athletic energy into the food for that coming week. Finding new recipes has become a delightful adventure. I confess, I never thought that would happen.

FIGURE OUT *YOUR* EATING PLAN

I describe what it took to revamp my eating plan, for a bit of inspiration and perhaps some motivation. Now it's your turn to take a look at your health as a whole. Consider your medical history, allergies, family history, current health conditions, and anything else that comes to mind in regard to your lifestyle and relationship with food. Then add them up to determine what food is best for you. A whole food, clean eating way of living does benefit nearly everyone, but that doesn't mean to be an athlete you need to be vegan and gluten-free. It's worth taking some time to figure out what works for you.

NUTRITION FOR AN ENDURANCE EVENT

Carbs

The body only has glycogen, which transforms into glucose, stored in the liver and muscles to cover about 90 minutes of exercise. So, for every training session I do that's over 90 minutes, I have to plan to feed my body carbohydrates, which is the exercising body's preferred form of fuel. This is especially important because of having type 1 diabetes. Carbs are sugars and starches that fuel our bodies much like gasoline fuels a race car. Each gram of carbohydrate contains about 4 calories worth of fuel. Just like a race car stores its fuel in a tank, the human body stores carbohydrates as glycogen in both our muscles and liver. These glycogen reserves are relied upon to stabilize blood sugars and allow for optimal muscle function.

The recommended amount of carbohydrates per hour for performance is 30 to 60 grams for women and up to 75 grams per hour for men. Having done a lot of trial-and-error experimentation, I've figured out that my ideal is 35 to 50 grams per hour. This varies somewhat by how well I've trained that season, and how fast I am attempting to go. Coach Nicole (who doesn't have diabetes) has often said to me, "When in doubt on a long ride, and you need extra power and energy, eat more!"

The amount that I need per hour is in addition to any glucose that I, as someone who has diabetes, needs for low blood sugars. It's important not to count glucose taken for lows in the totals I need per hour. I carry glucose tabs or Smarties on every ride and run and use those for low blood sugars, which can happen unexpectedly in an athletic event when you inject insulin.

For the carbs I use, I carry Honey Stinger, Huma and/or Gu gel packets, homemade dairy and gluten-free fig newtons, and Skratch Labs Exercise Hydration Mix. I also use dried mango and other dried fruit. These are quick carbs that are more natural, plus they taste good! Over the past few years, on my long runs and bike rides, I've started eating a packet of UCAN (which is a long-lasting superstarch) thirty minutes before I start the exercise session. Depending how many miles and hours I will be out there, I bring a few extra UCAN packets. UCAN works particularly well at stabilizing my energy and my glucose levels.

Before I go on a long training session and before event day, I spend time figuring out how I will carry all the carbs I'll need to eat. For cycling, I use a bento box (a box-like case that is mounted on the front bar of my bike) and I carry gels and fig newtons in my bike jersey. The many pockets in bike jerseys are helpful. I measure out the Skratch Labs mix into plastic baggies that I stash in my jersey and add it when I refill my water bottles. For running, I wear a Flipbelt that can store quite a bit of nutrition.

The thing to remember is that carbs fuel exercise and without them, you may suffer from fatigue and poor performance.

Hydration

In terms of hydration, it's important to drink at least one full water bottle per hour. Most bike water bottles hold about 24 ounces of liquid. Some are smaller, so I intentionally choose the larger water bottles. Hydration is critical for maintaining digestion. On the bike, one of the water bottles I carry is straight water, but the other bottle has Skratch Labs secret drink mix, which, the way I mix it, has about 30 grams of carbs in it. If it's particularly hot and humid, I make sure I have salt tablets or Nuun electrolyte tablets with me. I put those in my straight water bottle.

For long runs, I make sure to map out water stops. Occasionally, when running alone, I've driven the route in my car and dropped full water bottles behind a tree along the route I will run. I do this so I will have water as I'm doing that run.

In addition to the nutrition I carry with me, when running I always have a Flipbelt 10-ounce flat water bottle in my side pocket of my shorts or run pants. On the bike, I carry two water bottles and extra cash so that I can buy more water in case I can't find any free water on the route.

Train Your Stomach

One of the coaches I worked with defines an endurance athletic event as being one for which you have to eat in order to finish. I love this definition. Learning how to consume food while swimming a longer distance (3+ miles), biking, running, cross-country skiing and more is not easy. In addition to learning how to get nutrition into your body, you must train your stomach and digestive system how to process and digest it.

One bike ride I was on handed out food products at the rest stop that I had never eaten before. Toward the end of the ride, as I was pushing my body hard, all of a sudden my stomach revolted. That had never happened in a race. I had to stop my bike. I was afraid I would have diarrhea, but instead I grabbed my stomach and hurled everything I had eaten. It was ugly. The experience imprinted on my mind to never eat something during a race that I hadn't given my body a chance to practice digesting.

This is why almost all athletic events—and races—tell you in advance on their websites what nutrition and hydration products they plan to serve at their event. Pay attention to these announcements, and either bring your own, or practice with what they will offer. Please, don't surprise your digestive system on race/event day.

Hitting "The Wall" or Bonking

If you don't calculate your nutrition correctly for a long endurance event or training session, you will likely hit the wall, which is also known as bonking. This rarely ever happens to me because I pay such close attention to my nutrition due to having type 1 diabetes. Paying attention to my blood sugar during an event causes me to tune into what I am or am not eating, which saves me from bonking. That said, I've witnessed other athletes hitting the metaphorical wall, and let's just say it doesn't look pretty. Essentially, it's when the body runs out of nutritional resources.

The TrainerRoad blog, by Sean Hurley, describes bonking this way:

> It's a total inability to continue, marked by nausea, extreme physical weakness, poor coordination, and a profoundly awful feeling. Essentially, bonking is

exercise-induced hypoglycemia or low blood sugar. Typically, bonking is preceded by waves of progressively worsening symptoms.

At first, you may feel hungry or exhibit negative self-talk that eventually leads to an increase in your rate of perceived exertion (RPE). As a bonk gets worse, you may develop a headache, nausea, shaking hands, loss of focus, or dizziness. If the bonking continues, so does the likelihood of confusion and the inability to function physically.[3]

Learn your body and practice your event-day nutrition.

Why Eating Clean Ahead of an Event Is Critical

Coach Nicole Freedman taught me the value of controlling everything possible in the week before a big event. The big event is often referred to as your "A-Race," meaning this is the event you have trained for all season. You can't control the weather or the training time that has already passed. Rather than fret about what the weather will be or whether or not you did enough or too much training, in that week before your event or race, you *can* control the food you put into your body. Granted, you can control the food you put into your body during all your training weeks; but for sure, that week leading up to an important race, it's valuable to eat as clean as you possibly can.

In my case, that means I minimize the processed food even more than I usually do. I make a concerted effort to increase the variety and quantity of vegetables I'm eating. I don't eat sugary desserts. I eliminate all animal products, including eggs and cheese, which I sometimes eat these days. I rarely eat out, and the week before an A-Race event, I make a pointed effort to not eat out at all. After all, it's quite difficult to control the items a restaurant puts into the food when you eat out. I make sure I'm eating enough calories every day, so that the glycogen in my liver and muscles is fully stocked up, since I'm going to pull on that supply on race day. I've noticed over the years that eating so carefully and intentionally the week to ten days before race day feels good. It acts like a reminder to my whole system of how good it feels to eat with purpose and focus.

WEIGHT LOSS AND ENDURANCE ATHLETICS

Losing weight is a complicated topic. Each of us is very different. Many consider weight loss to be all about "eat fewer calories and move your body more." I wish it was that simple. In my case, it took going on the drug Ozempic to help me lose the weight that crept up on me. Working with a registered dietitian who also understood endurance athletics and diabetes made all the difference. In recent years, Ozempic has gotten a lot of attention in the news as a weight-loss drug. It does help me keep my weight down, but the reason it helped me lose weight is because, as a person with type 1 diabetes, I'm missing other hormones besides insulin. I'm missing the hormone that tells me I'm full. Ozempic gives that hormone back to me and now when I eat, I actually feel full. Turns out satiety helps me stop eating.

One thing I keep in mind these days, as I now feel good in my body after many years of hard work, is that muscle does weigh more than fat. My current weight is 154 pounds and I'm 5 feet 6 inches tall. I used to think my ideal weight was

145 pounds, but that was before I consistently lifted weights. Worst of all, that number wasn't based on anything logical. It was some made up number that I thought would be a "perfect" weight. Instead, what I've learned is that loving this body, and all the amazing things it is capable of doing, is the bigger win.

Losing weight while training for a race or event can be quite difficult to do. Mainly because when you're eating to lose pounds, you aren't eating for athletic performance. Weight loss and athletic performance are different ways to focus your eating energy. When I've wanted to drop some pounds, I've worked on that in my "off-season" (the time of year when I'm not training for a specific event or race). That makes it easier to focus on eating to lose pounds.

In short, if your goal is to lose weight, I strongly encourage you to get support to make that happen.

POST-EXERCISE RECOVERY FUELING

My last comment about nutrition and endurance exercise is all about the importance of recovery fueling. There are entire books about this topic. My guidance is to be sure to fuel your body temple with healthy food after you complete a big athletic training or event. This is especially true for any session lasting longer than 90 minutes. Your muscles and organs need to be replenished.

If possible, eat some good calories in the 45 to 60 minutes after you finish your exercise session. This hour is referred to as the "Golden Hour" because it is when the body most effectively absorbs nutrients, and glycogen is replaced very efficiently since it was just depleted.[4] I make an effort to eat a good balance of protein and healthy carbohydrates during this Golden Hour.

Eat well. You are worth it. Chances are good you'll notice how good you feel when you make smart nutrition choices.

TRY THIS

Journal

Get your journal and reflect on what you ate during the past 24 hours. No one will look at this list except you, so be 100 percent honest. After you do this, write about your relationship with food. Are you happy with how you eat? Are you unhappy?

Write down one or two very specific things you could do to improve your athletic nutrition. Is there anyone you want to consult with about your eating? Who might that person be?

Notes

1. See Kris Carr at http://kriscarr.com.
2. See Brendan Brazier at https://myvega.com/about-us/brendan-brazier.
3. "What is Bonking? Causes, Dangers and Prevention," Sean Hurley, TrainerRoad, accessed August 28, 2023, https://www.trainerroad.com/blog/what-is-bonking-causes-dangers-and-prevention.
4. See "The Best Post-Workout Fuel," Carmen Roberts, HealthCentral, July 25, 2016, https://www.healthcentral.com/article/the-best-postworkout-fuel.

Resources

Rules of endurance eating: http://www.ironman.com/triathlon-news/articles/2013/06/6-rules-of-endurance-nutrition.aspx#axzz4tWz9wwCx

More about eating right for endurance: http://www.eatright.org/resource/fitness/training-and-recovery/endurance-and-cardio/eat-right-for-endurance

Nutrition for endurance athletes: https://www.trainingpeaks.com/blog/nutrition-for-endurance-athletes-101/#

Carol LeCroy: https://www.acupunctureplus.net

T. Colin Campbell, PhD: http://nutritionstudies.org

Marcey Robinson, MS, RD, CSSD, BC-ADM: http://achievehp.com

12 Ways to Eat Healthy No Matter How Busy You Are: https://www.entrepreneur.com/article/245770#

Clean Eating: http://www.cookinglight.com/eating-smart/smart-choices/clean-eating

Paleo Lo-Carb for Endurance Athletes: http://www.stack.com/a/the-paleo-diet-for-endurance-athletes-a-guide-to-training-without-carbs

Good book about how to incorporate fasting into your life: *Fast Like a Girl: A Woman's Guide to Using the Healing Power of Fasting to Burn Fat, Boost Energy, and Balance Hormones* by Dr. Mindy Pelz.

Products Mari Uses

Skratch Labs https://www.skratchlabs.com

UCAN https://ucan.co

Nuun electrolyte tablets https://nuunlife.com

Honey Stinger https://honeystinger.com

Gu gels https://guenergy.com

Huma gels https://humagel.com

CHAPTER 9

SLEEP AND RECOVERY MATTER

"A good laugh and a long sleep are the
best cures in the doctor's book."

—*IRISH PROVERB*

MY CYCLING COACH, NICOLE FREEDMAN, IS ONE OF THE best sleep experts I've ever met. Hanging out with her at endurance athlete camps, I would watch her fall asleep in the back of the room. She did this because she loves napping and every time we fall asleep, our bodies generate muscle-repair hormones. Of course, at the time I watched her fall asleep, I didn't know this; and until I talked to her about it, I thought she was sleep deprived or maybe just super bored with the presentation topic. Turns out she's for sure not sleep deprived, and while she was generally very well versed in the topics being covered, she was rarely bored. She simply highly valued napping.

When Nicole was racing professionally and visited me in Colorado (when I was going through chemo and radiation), she'd jump for joy that I needed to go to bed by 8:00 p.m. because I was so exhausted from the treatments. Nicole's idea of a good 24-hour period is if she can sleep for 9 to 12 hours of it. Given how low sleep is on the list of priorities for many of us, I was impressed that Nicole put sleep at nearly the top of her list of things to take care of.

After my second bout of cancer, I realized that I had managed to develop cancer twice, and thus I needed to examine all aspects of my life and modify where I could and had control. Once was bad; twice was a big wake-up call. I needed to seriously review what I could control in my life and change what I could. In addition to changing how I ate every day, another top item was how much rest and relaxation I allowed myself.

Before becoming an endurance athlete, I had spent a fair amount of time in therapy for the sexual abuse I survived as a child. I'd learned that one of the ways to reset my nervous system and allow my spirit to recover from the memory process was by sleeping. I've struggled for most of my life with being able to fall asleep and stay asleep for more than three or four hours at a time. Thankfully, as I continued doing various kinds of therapy, especially inner child healing and somatic healing such as TRE[2], my sleeping has gotten better. Turns out, sleep is healing and rejuvenating. This is especially true for older endurance athletes, like me.

RECORD-KEEPING FOR ATHLETES

When I started hanging out with Chris Klebl, he, like Nicole Freedman, was obsessed with sleep, knowing as he did that sleep allowed his body critical time to recover from the stress of intensive workouts. Chris recorded in a little notebook exactly what training he did every day, what he ate, and how many hours he slept. As someone who has type 1 diabetes and, thus, values record-keeping, watching Chris woke me up to the realization that keeping track of things is super helpful. Not just people with chronic health conditions keep records. Chris and Nicole were onto something.

THE PURPOSE OF SLEEP

It's easy in our work-hard-play-hard world to forget why sleep is important. Perhaps like me you've heard countless people say, "I'll sleep when I'm dead." I was talking to a new friend who bragged about how she functioned "just fine" on five hours of sleep a night. (She was hoping to do a 100-mile bike ride with me a few summers ago.)

During sleep, your body cycles through several stages throughout the night, alternating between non-rapid eye movement and rapid eye movement. Although growth and repair occur throughout all the stages, rapid eye movement stages have the greatest release of the growth hormones, which promotes protein synthesis and tissue growth and repair.

Insufficient sleep leads to increased levels of stress-related hormones such as cortisol, plus catecholamines in the blood, impairing muscle recovery. If you have a chronic sleep deficit during training, your body may not be able to recover suffi-ciently between training sessions, compromising your ability to train hard. Additionally, this combination of sleep deprivation and hard training will eventually put you in an overtrained state and reduce performance.

All the best endurance training programs I've followed promote a weekly rhythm of work, work, work, rest. This type of plan is called periodization. Learning to navigate a rest week was a big task for me. Growing up in a dysfunctional family, I fell into the belief that staying busy and active all the time was the way to win love, avoid conflict, and succeed. In my case, as a young child I noticed that my mother kept busy all the time. She insisted that I stay busy all the time too. As I grew up, and was in high school then college, I had integrated this belief that my value was only as good as how much I was contributing to the world around me. Simply put, my value was based on how busy I was. In high school, I was in more than three clubs and organizations at all of the high schools I attended. I attended three different high schools over the four years of high school. This was another symptom of my desperate desire to fit in and belong. I kept moving around hoping that eventually I would find a place that I fit, and that I mattered. At all three schools, I was in many different clubs and organizations, often rising to positions of leadership. In my senior year of high school, I was a yearbook editor and the student council president. Plus, I had a part-time job that I got when I was fifteen years old. Being busy was the way to be accepted, approved of, and valued in my family.

This pattern of behavior continued through college. In fact, I remember my younger brother driving me to an activist gathering when I was very sick with a cold, saying to me, "You know, if you're sick and exhausted, not only are you harming yourself, you really can't be of much use to anyone you're trying to motivate at this meeting." I remember thinking to myself, "What do you know? Being involved and busy is the only way to belong and matter." Little did I understand at the time how much I was hurting myself.

Take a moment and reflect about your relationship with sleep and rest. Does it come easy for you to get enough sleep? Do you have any patterns in your life that might be helpful to change as you become an endurance athlete? A key thing to understand is that you will perform better and overall feel better if you can incorporate healthy sleep routines into your life.

THERMOREGULATION

In my quest to improve my sleep behavior, I studied sleep hygiene. I'm not a scientist, but I do enjoy reading science information. In addition to my sleep challenges, my body doesn't handle heat very well, in part because I'm not that good at sweating. Sweating is an important thing the body does to cool down when it's hot. Turns out lack of sleep reduces the body's ability to dissipate heat during exercise. As you might imagine, that too can hurt your endurance performance. Thermoregulation is what the body does to maintain a stable core temperature. Sweating is one way the body maintains temperature equilibrium.

"A study published in the 'American Journal of Physiology' showed that sleep-deprived, endurance-trained men had a higher esophageal temperature and sweated less in response to cycling in a warm room compared to when they were well-rested, indicating the lack of sleep reduced their ability to regulate body temperature. Lack of sleep could cause your race performance to suffer, particularly in hot weather. Yet another reason getting sufficient sleep is critical."[2]

NIGHTTIME ROUTINE

I've never been much of a television watcher, so I've never had a television or computer in my bedroom. Turns out, that helps. I always sleep with a lightweight blanket over my eyes which conveniently blocks all light, again making it easier to fall asleep, and stay asleep. I've also developed a few routines I do every night to signal to my body and mind that bedtime and sleep time is near. I flip my day-calendar to the next day and read with thoughtfulness the quote by Louise Hay who always offers a wise mantra for the coming day. Next, I walk over to my wall calendar and select a sticker that represents how the day went. I love stickers. Super silly, and that's okay. It reminds my adult self to be playful and lighthearted. The stickers often make me chuckle, and putting the sticker on for that day signals to my inner self that I successfully survived that day. The small act of sticking that sticker on the calendar is another signal to my subconscious that the day is done, and it's time to let go.

Then I climb into bed and pull out my Gratitude Journal. I take a few deep breaths and select a colorful marker and think about all the amazing things that happened to me that day. I have the expectation that wondrous things will happen to me every day, and miraculously, since that's what I expect, that is in fact what happens. As I write down at least ten things I'm grateful for that day, it allows me to drift back into recalling all the joy, love, and delight that happened. Some days I'm struck with the magic I experienced at the freshness of the air, the bright diamond sunlight reflection on the lake I ran by, or the peacefulness of walking a few miles with my dog. The best part of my Gratitude Journal reflection is that it reminds me of all the abundance and love in my life. After closing the journal, I turn off the light and snuggle down into the bed. I put on my Perytong wireless sleep headphones headband[3] and I select one of the sleep meditations on the Insight Timer app on my phone. I breathe slowly and deeply and tell my inner child self that I am safe and secure and now it's time to sleep. With luck and good fortune, I get 8 to 9 hours of solid sleep every night. In my case, that much sleep is essential for restoring my mental acuity and helping my body recover from the exercise session(s) I did that day (and plan to do the next day).

Now that I'm in my late fifties, I finally understand how important consistent, deep sleep of at least 8 hours a night is. One of the most amazing side effects of the somatic, inner child healing I've done slowly over time with the help of many different, wise therapists, is that I finally can sleep more than five hours without waking up. I still usually get up at least once during the night to pee and resettle, but thankfully, I finally feel safe and secure in my own body and being, and I can sleep a whole night. Not any coincidence, I suspect that plays a role in me getting faster with my biking and running. Good, solid sleep, strength training, clean eating, and interval workouts in combination have made me a better athlete as a middle-aged person, compared to when I was just getting started as an endurance athlete in my thirties.

Take a moment to consider your nighttime routine. Do you have one? Could you modify it to make it more effective for you?

RECOVERY

As our bodies age, you may have noticed that the recovery ability you had when you were younger seems to fade. In fact, in recent years, recovery has become a hot topic in the world of endurance athletics. I'm a low-budget athlete, so I like to do recovery that fits in my budget. There are many things you too can do to help your body recover and heal from exercise sessions. You might be surprised about how many options there are for you.

Sleep is one part of the rest and recovery equation. Recovery includes a few other activities too. As I age and continue to love endurance sports, I find that recovery is not only good for me, it helps keep me healthy and in a good mood. In other words, recovery activities are good for the body and the mind. Listed below are the recovery activities I use, which are acupuncture, massage, chiropractic care, physical therapy, yoga, and meditation.

Acupuncture

I discovered acupuncture when I lived in Santa Cruz, California. I was in my mid-twenties, and I was still suffering from debilitating headaches. I didn't know why. I felt all kinds of pressure in the front of my forehead and behind my face. Turns out I had sinus issues. In those days I was eating quite a lot of dairy products. A friend suggested I try acupuncture. Since I have diabetes, and at that time I was giving myself four to six shots a day, the needles of acupuncture didn't bother me. My health insurance covered the cost, so I found an acupuncturist and I went. The first needles that Nancy put in my face were like magic. Nearly miraculously the needles released the pressure in my face and head. Nancy kept putting needles in my feet, my ears, and on my hands. I felt my whole body relax and settle.

Since then, I've managed to go to acupuncture two to three times a month since I discovered it. Turns out there are trained and licensed acupuncturists in all major cities in the United States. Acupuncture was a lifesaver when I was going through cancer treatments.

One of the acupuncturists I met when I lived in Colorado was Whitfield Reaves. He was an instructor at Southwest Acupuncture College that offered free acupuncture to those who were cancer survivors. Whit had been a team acupuncturist in the 1980s for the USA Olympic marathon run team and understands sports recovery well. At that time, Whit was working on what would be an important book in the sports acupuncture world, *The Acupuncture Handbook of Sports Injuries and Pain.*

At that point in my athletic career, I was having a difficult time running longer than three miles without pain. Meaning that at two and a half miles, my right leg would start to have sharp pain in the muscle along the bone in the front of my lower leg. At three miles the pain routinely became excruciating, and I would have to walk and discontinue the run. Whit taught the student acupuncturists how to thread a needle in my front calf. It was amazing and caused the muscles and energy in my body to move freely. Whit also tracked the lower leg pain up to my hip and glutes. After a few sessions, Whit suggested I visit a Boulder sports clinic for an assessment. I went and their analysis, which Whit had suspected, was that I had a weak butt. Thankfully, a weak butt can be made stronger. With regularity, I do several Jane Fonda butt strengthening exercises, namely leg lifts where I focus on my butt muscles, because keeping my butt strong requires consistent effort.

Whit also told me that the pain in my lower leg might never fully resolve and that to continue to be a runner might require regular acupuncture. That continues to be true. These days here in Minnesota, I have found another acupuncturist that I see three times a month. John Falls puts needles in my legs, hips, and glutes nearly every session, and these days I run with nearly zero pain as a result. It's worth all the time and money to make this a recovery part of my athletic routine.

Have you ever tried acupuncture? If so, how was it?

Massage

I discovered massage when I lived in Hilton Head Island in South Carolina one college summer. A friend of mine was enrolled in a certification program and they needed people to practice on. I said sure, not really knowing what professional massage was all about. I was immediately hooked. Every massage I get (I go for at least one every month), I find myself tuning into the wisdom of my body. The quiet, the kind caring, and the safe touch all combine to allow my whole self to deeply relax and let go. I find that I breathe more smoothly, and I can feel my cortisol levels lower. Plus, my tense shoulders and tense muscles everywhere in my body let go. Over the years I've discovered that getting a massage a few days before a big event or race actually helps me perform better. I strongly recommend massage as a recovery strategy. Give it a try!

Chiropractic Care

When I lived in Santa Cruz and was doing intensive mental health therapy, I experienced lots of physical pain as my body released many years of bottled-up trauma and pain that I had stuffed down. It helped that I had discovered acupuncture. I kept searching for more relief, and I found a chiropractor I liked. Turns out my spine is curved—I don't quite have scoliosis, but almost. In addition, I fell off a fence in a trust building exercise (the irony doesn't escape me) at a diabetes camp I was working at in California. The fall hurt my neck and shoulder. Additionally, I have a tendency to jut my chin forward when

I'm working at a computer or simply moving in life. In combination, these injuries and body behaviors make me a good candidate for chiropractic care. After Santa Cruz and going to that early chiropractor, I took some time off from chiropractic care. Then about a year ago, I noticed a clicking sound in my right hip socket. It scared me and made me wonder if I was going to damage my hip and need hip surgery or a hip replacement. It's true, I can be a bit of a hypochondriac.

My Inner Healer suggested I give chiropractic another chance. I did a search of near-to-my-house, covered-by-my-health-insurance chiropractors and found Life Force chiropractic, with Dr. Sadie Knickrehm. Dr. Sadie is herself an athlete and right away she figured out things to do with my hip and leg that made the clicking stop. She gave me a few exercises to do and so far, so good. Much better than hip surgery or some other extreme solution. Even better, Dr. Sadie has a running background, and my work with her is helping my running get stronger and faster. A total win! If you can figure out a way to fit chiropractic recovery into your life, I would encourage it.

Physical Therapy

I've had a few injuries along the way. (I've broken my ankle twice, and I've had to have trigger finger surgery on three different fingers.) In these instances, physical therapy helped my recovery go more smoothly—and, I think, faster. The PTs (physical therapists) I worked with understood the body and the healing process with precision. They gave me exercises to do and they were supportive as my body healed. In the event you should injure yourself, please seek support from everyone you believe will be helpful. Include physical therapy if you can.

Yoga

When I lived in Santa Cruz, I discovered the joy of yoga. This was back when I had a lot of physical pain from the sexual abuse I was healing from and old, stored physical trauma was coming to the surface. This was when I found acupuncture and chiropractic to help my body move through that early pain. Yoga was another modality that taught me to slow down and notice what was happening in my body as I moved. There are many varieties of yoga, and my suggestion is to see which type speaks to you.

These days I do five simple yoga poses nearly every evening before climbing into bed to sleep. The poses are Uttanasana (Standing Forward Bend), Supta Baddha Konasana (Reclining Bound Angle), Balasana (Child's Pose), Reclining Spinal Twist, and one of my all-time favorites, Viparita Karani (Legs Up the Wall.)[4] I found this series in *Yoga Journal* and doing the poses each evening helps me sleep. If you could use a bit more help with sleep, give this series a try and see if it helps you.

Meditation

As I've mentioned throughout this book, meditation has been a life-saving practice for me. Teaching myself how to follow my breath and to observe my thinking as I have thoughts has taught me how to slow down and find self-love and peace within my being.

That first meditation retreat I did with Jack Kornfield (where he asked me and all the participants to practice being quiet for a full day) was the launch into my more than twenty-two-year everyday meditation practice. When I was in the psychiatric hospital after my suicide attempt in 2013, one person who I talked to on the phone a few times for support and hope was meditation teacher and guiding leader of Common Ground Meditation Center in Minneapolis, Minnesota, Mark Nunberg. Mark reminded me to practice meditation in the hospital as much as I could. His suggestion is potentially what saved me from having dramatic brain damage from the suicide attempt. For a few weeks, the doctors were concerned that I might never regain enough brain function to ever hold another job, to drive a car, or to live alone. They noticed that I struggled to form complete words and sentences. It was a rough few weeks.

Then I talked to Mark, and something inside me remembered that I knew how to sit in meditation practice. There was a lot of unstructured time in that psychiatric ward. They had random groups we could attend, and various arts and crafts classes we could participate in, but they weren't required. They didn't want patients to sleep excessively, but I figured out sitting in meditation baffled them. Within a few days, they realized I was not sleeping, and I was not disturbing anyone, and they let me be.

For about twenty days in a row, I sat in meditation practice for at least six hours a day. I focused on my breathing, and I tuned into what was happening within me at that moment. I simply paid attention to my thoughts and my body. At the moments I got frustrated with the hospital and my situation in the hospital, I again would slow myself down, pay attention to my breathing, and notice that in that moment I was safe, I had enough food, and I had myself, and this meditation practice. I took refuge in knowing that for many centuries monks have sat in meditation for hours upon hours. I was in good company sitting on the floor on a pillow on a towel in my hospital room with my back straight. I don't have any proof that all that meditation made a difference, but I believe that if nothing else, it didn't hurt my recovery process.

I continue my daily meditation practice now, and I suspect I will until my last day here. Taking 10 to 30 minutes a day allows my entire being to slow down, reset, and relax. Helpful skills in this stress-filled life. Please consider giving meditation a try.

Fun

Another key to successful recovery is laughter and enjoyment of life. Seems obvious, I know. In my case, remembering to schedule activities just for the fun of them takes a bit of effort. I don't enjoy big crowds, so music festivals and bars aren't enjoyable anymore. I didn't mind these sorts of venues when I was younger and less attuned to where in the world I felt safe and secure. As a result, these days the activities that feel most fun and relaxing are taking my dog to the dog park or meeting up with a friend or two for a home-cooked meal. Thankfully, long slow runs and summertime bike rides and swimming at the lake are great opportunities to meet up with good people, share lots of laughter, and spin delightful stories together. The key is to schedule fun. Remember you are worth it. Your athletic body and soul will thank you for the down time with friends.

TRY THIS

Journal

Step 1: Write about how much sleep you get a night. Describe your sleep routine. Do you have any sleep challenges? If so, what are they? Have you ever gotten any support about your sleep challenges? If yes, from whom and was it helpful? If you've never gotten support for your sleep challenges, who could you consult now? Write down their name and make a plan to reach out.

Step 2: Continue in your journal, reflecting on the additional rest and recovery activities that work for you. Have you tried acupuncture, massage, or chiropractic? Why or why not? Are you open to finding this sort of care? What about meditation and fun? Do you make time for these in your life? What resistance or willingness do you notice?

Notes

1. Somatic healing and TRE, https://traumaprevention.com.
2. "The Effects of Sleep on Performance in Endurance Athletes," Gina Battaglia, azcentral., accessed August 29, 2023, http://healthyliving.azcentral.com/effects-sleep-performance-endurance-athletes-3628.html.
3. Perytong wireless sleep headphones from Amazon: https://amzn.to/3DsrGGQ.
4. See "5 Simple Stretches to Help You Sleep Better (That You Can Do in Less Than 10 Minutes)," Jessica Conner, Yoga Journal, March 11, 2022, https://www.yogajournal.com/poses/yoga-by-benefit/insomnia/5-yoga-stretches-to-help-you-sleep-better.

5. Common Ground Meditation Center in Minneapolis, MN: https://commongroundmeditation.org.

Resources

Bright Spots & Landmines: The Diabetes Guide I Wish Someone Had Handed Me by Adam Brown

The Sleep Revolution: Transforming Your Life, One Night at a Time by Arianna Huffington

Whitfield Reaves: https://www.whitfieldreaves.com

CHAPTER 10

TRAINING PLANS

"I am building a fire, and every day I train
I am adding more fuel."

—MIA HAMM

IN PART BECAUSE OF HAVING HAD DIABETES FOR MORE than forty years, I have no illusion that I can show up to a half-marathon or an 80-mile bike ride or even a sprint distance triathlon without having done training for the event. I'm grateful that, other than the very first triathlon I did in 2005, I've always done at least some intentional training to prepare both my mind and my body to perform as well as possible. I strongly encourage you to do the same.

Once you have selected your race or event, it's time to find a training program. This might take some research and strategy, but you are smart, and you can figure it out.

Answering these four questions will help you figure out what steps you can take to train for your athletic event. Take a bit of time to get accurate answers. Write down the questions and answers in your journal under the name and date of the event you plan to do.

CHAPTER 10: TRAINING PLANS

QUESTION 1: HOW MUCH TIME DO
I HAVE BEFORE MY EVENT?

Figure out in terms of weeks how much time you have before your next event to make sure you have enough time to get solidly trained. For a 100-mile bike ride, for instance, I like to have 18 weeks to train. For a sprint triathlon, I schedule 12–14 weeks of training. Weeks are a good way to think about time in terms of endurance athletics, and most training plans put together by highly qualified coaches are organized this way. In my case, I appreciate the weeks format because going into the training I can easily visualize how long I have to get my body and mind ready for the event.

For shorter distance events (such as a sprint distance triathlon, a 5K run race, or a 25–35-mile bike event), I strongly recommend at least 12 weeks to get yourself trained and ready. That said, once you gain fitness in one sport, it will translate to fitness in other sports and you might not need quite as many weeks to get yourself ready.

QUESTION 2: HOW MUCH MONEY DO
I HAVE TO SPEND ON TRAINING?

Good coaching isn't cheap. I owned a company that trained people with diabetes to be endurance athletes and, as a result, did quite a bit of research about the going rates. At the time I owned TeamWILD Athletics LLC, we charged a flat fee of $500 for our 18-week programs. Granted, our programs had athletic coaching and diabetes coaching, which combined a number of resources for our participants. Not many programs combine like that.

A few years ago, I had a half-marathon I was doing, and I used Jeff Galloway's run-walk-run training program.[1] The program is a 17-week program that suggested I run three to four times a week for 17 weeks. I've read a few of Galloway's books, and I found his app (which is available on the Apple App Store). For what you get, it's not a very expensive app. What I appreciate about the app is that it gave me a very clear training plan for 17 weeks that made me confident and ready to complete the half-marathon, which I did with success. In fact, it was such a good half-marathon, I put two in my plan for the next year. This time I joined Run Minnesota, which resulted in gaining access to three outstanding endurance running coaches.

Here in Minnesota there's an organization called Run Minnesota[2] and they train people for half-marathons and full marathons. To join the training group costs a little over $200. CTS Train Right training programs offer coaching in a wide variety of sports including cycling, ultrarunning, and triathlon at a minimum of $197 per month. You get custom-for-you coaching by licensed and certified coaches. CTS is based in Colorado, and they offer their services to athletes worldwide.

Another great resource for those of you who are triathletes is to join USAT, which is USA Triathlon. Once you are a member (it costs about $50 annually) you gain access to more than 20 free training plans created by more than 18 certified coaches. These plans are not custom directly to you, but they are good, and will get you there.

In essence, coaching is an investment that's worth it. That said, many times you can find good beginner programs online for little to no cost. I've provided a few training resources at chapter's end in the Resources section.

QUESTION 3: WHAT GEAR DO I NEED FOR THE EVENT?

I went into gear in detail in chapter 7, please refer to that section for more info. I have gear here again, because having the right gear will give you so much confidence as you approach your event. Silly, I know, but gear does matter. Ideally, get as specific as possible about the gear you'll need for the event you've signed up to do.

Another thing to think about is given how many weeks you will be training; will your gear requirements change as the weeks go by? For example, when I have big cycling events and run events that will happen in the summer, but I start training when there's snow on the ground, and it's super cold here in Minnesota. I'm not a winter cyclist, yet anyway, so my wintertime cycling happens on a bike trainer that holds my bike in the basement or in a spare room or space. Acquiring the proper gear, not just to participate in the event, but to prepare for it as well, will make the training easier and bolster your motivation as you get out and train.

QUESTION 4: WHO AMONG MY FRIENDS AND FAMILY COULD I TRAIN WITH?

I went into detail about friends and family to train with in chapter 6, so please refer to that chapter for more depth about why it's so important to have people to do your event and the training alongside. I've done a number of big events alone, including doing most of the training alone. Training alone is beautiful; I find it meditative, a chance to be inside my own head and access my spirit.

Yet training alone is hard. For me it's hard because there are days when I get lazy and unmotivated and if the only person who cares that I make it to my training session is me, it's easy to not do it. Accountability to just yourself isn't simple. There are some people who have no trouble with getting out for every workout session by themselves. I used to think that was me, but over time, I've realized friends and teammates make a major positive difference. Some days it's just knowing one friend is counting on me showing up that will get me out there.

Once on Christmas, I was essentially alone for the whole day, and I dragged myself out to run by the Mississippi River where I often do training runs with my athletic friends. Running on the familiar route made it easy to pretend that I was running with my friends. I knew they would be happy that I got out there to train. As I finished up the run, I unexpectedly passed one of the women from my Thursday morning run interval class. Meg called out, "Merry Christmas, Mari!" I called out the same to her. Just seeing her on the route brought a huge smile to my face and reminded me that even though I was alone on Christmas, I wasn't lonely. In fact, not only was I not lonely, I belonged and people noticed I was alive and well. Given my background, these unexpected, joyful reminders mean the world.

Therefore, it helps to find friends and/or family members to train with and maybe even do an event together. The biggest benefit is accountability. Plus, it makes the whole thing more fun. After all, there's at least one person who cares that you show up to train and at least one person at the event to be there with you at the finish line to celebrate the accomplishment.

MAKE IT REAL

Once you've answered the above four questions, now it's time to put your training plan into action. Taking action means moving from the theoretical realm of planning and thinking about your event, into the practical, actionable realm of daily practice. Now you will start moving your body and mind in the direction of being able to show up at your event ready to perform.

I've been called audacious, which is another way to say bold and plucky. By choosing to call yourself an athlete, setting a goal, finding a training plan, and perhaps engaging a coach, you too, are audacious and plucky. I hope you smile imagining yourself as audacious.

You get to make your vision real, which means taking steps to make it a reality. Once the planning is done, here are the things I do when I start training for a big event. I like to call events "big," because doing so creates importance in my mind. Making events important increases the sense of value in what you are doing.

Many coaches refer to athletic events as "A" or "B" or "C" events. Meaning that your A races are the main or big races that you are training for in that year. B and C races are still important races, but you don't develop your training plan around B and C events. These events are ideally intended to boost your confidence and sense of fun and enjoyment on your way to a solid performance at your A race/event.

Put All Your Workouts on Your Calendar

Taking action and making things real requires you to do a few things. I use a few methods to keep myself focused and forward moving. The first thing I do is use Google Calendar and create a dedicated training exercise calendar that's a different color than my normal life calendar. I can show just the exercise calendar or combine it with my full life calendar. Seeing this calendar helps me imagine my exercise sessions as an important part of my week and life.

A number of years ago I started making official appointments with myself to work out. I take the appointments I make with others seriously—they are important. However, for a lot of my life, I didn't take my appointments with myself seriously. In essence, I didn't value myself as much as I valued friends and colleagues. That shifted when I started calling myself an athlete. I realized if I wanted to take my athletic self seriously, I needed to prioritize my exercise plans. After I do a training session, I go back into my calendar, and I give myself an X and an exclamation point. The X! indicates to my subconscious self that the session mattered, and I accomplished it. Often in the notes section of the calendar entry, I will jot down exactly what I did for that session and how I felt doing it.

If I'm being super on top of it, I will also note the weather conditions. Turns out weather does impact both training and performance at events. For example, we burn more calories when we run outside in extreme cold. I have to watch my blood sugar more carefully during the transition seasons, since my body has to acclimate. This is also true when I'm exercising in extreme humidity. Not that I burn more calories, but since I'm not that good at sweating, I have a difficult time with body temperature regulation, and I often get excessively dizzy if I haven't consumed enough electrolytes and sodium. As a result, over time I've learned the value of taking detailed notes about each exercise session, and then going back and reviewing them every few weeks and learning from both the mistakes and the successes I've had.

Do you keep a calendar for your work or personal life? If so, consider creating an exercise calendar for yourself. If you're a paper/pen calendar person, is there a way to add exercise to your system to make it happen for you?

Map Out Your Training for a Week or Two at a Time

This circles back to using your calendar and putting your workouts in said calendar. I do this every Sunday evening. I pay attention to my work and social calendar, and I figure out when I will do my workouts for the entire week. The items I put in my calendar, work, social, and exercise become top priority. Having them in my calendar makes it real.

This seems like an easy thing to do, but it took me a few years to get into the solid habit of doing this every single Sunday evening. It takes about fifteen minutes to plan and visualize what I will athletically do that coming week. I consider these fifteen minutes of scheduling, reviewing, and visualizing to be a focused, intention-setting block of time. By taking those minutes to visualize my week, it helps me commit to the plan I am setting up. It also reminds me of who I will see at each workout session. This reminds me that I'm accountable to myself and to my teammates and friends.

Print Out Your Full Training Plan

If you got your training plan from your coach or from an online program, print it all out. I have a friend who transcribes the program to a handwritten piece of paper, that's how helpful she finds the process to be. You want to see the full scope of what you've committed to doing. Read and review the full training plan. For example, since I used a 17-week Jeff Galloway app for my half-marathon training program, the full program is embedded in the app. I took an hour and scrolled through each of the training sessions in the app for all 17 weeks and wrote them down. I even went so far as to type them up so that I would have the entire training plan in front of me in black and white for easy review and study.

Noticing the plan's duration and what you'll be doing each week is helpful with visualization and a deeper understanding of where you're headed. When I trained to do the Half Ironman in Austin, Texas, I committed to doing nine workout sessions a week, which meant some double days and brick workouts. Double days are when you do one workout in the morning and another at lunch or after work. Bricks are when you do two sports back-to-back, the end result being that, after biking and running, your legs feel like bricks. Fitting in nine workouts in six days is a challenge. I say six days because having a scheduled rest day is critical. In my case, since I have a dog, I did an active recovery day and walked my dog at the time, Mack.

Seeing your full training regimen at the start of your training and then periodically reviewing where you are will again bolster your sense of accomplishment. You want to make your training plan yours, and having it visually in front of you will help that happen.

When You Finish Each Training Session, Mark It Off and Celebrate

In the Google calendar I note how many hours I exercised for each session I complete and give myself that X and that exclamation point to indicate that I did it and that I celebrated that

I did it. These small, consistent reminders of my success and strength pay off on race day by giving myself a boost in confidence. This simple act is a mini celebration.

Figure out a system of acknowledgement and simple celebration that will work for you. This will help keep you motivated and inspired as you train for your event.

Celebrate Your First Success

When I start training for a 100-mile bike ride, I make sure to celebrate my very first workout session using rewards that mean something to me. One of my favorite celebrations is to schedule a massage. Being able to relax and have my sore muscles rubbed for an hour is a heavenly way to celebrate a big accomplishment (starting a training program *is* an important accomplishment). I for sure take a selfie and post my success on social media. Other things I do to celebrate are to buy a new book or some music I've wanted. Sometimes I do something simple, like put on good tunes and dance around smiling: the original Happy Dance. I say again and again to myself, "I am worth celebrating! You are worth celebrating!" Accomplishing a major event is cause for celebration and delight.

Once you've answered the above four questions (chosen a training plan, hired a coach, found a team, and recruited a friend or two), be sure you do one quick happy dance and give yourself a high five! I am very proud of you for making this happen. You are taking charge of your health and wellness.

TRY THIS

Journal

Take a moment and write down ideas you have for finding a training plan for your event. Does the event you've signed up for offer training plans? If yes, is the plan detailed enough upon review to get you to the finish line with confidence? If not, where else can you find resources? Spend some time thinking of all your resources. Then go find them. Keep reminding yourself that the universe wants to support you and opening yourself to find what you need will happen.

Take a moment now to figure out how many weeks you have from today until your event. Once you know with clarity exactly how many weeks, does this time frame give you confidence that you have time to train for your event, or does it make you nervous? If it makes you nervous, think of what you can do to settle yourself and get support.

Notes

1. Jeff Galloway, http://www.jeffgalloway.com
2. Run Minnesota, https://www.run-minnesota.org/join

Resources

TriDot Training: https://tridot.com
HeartZones Training: https://www.heartzones.com
Beginner Triathlete: https://beginnertriathlete.com
USAT: https://www.usatriathlon.org
USATF: https://www.usatf.org
TrainRight coaching support: https://trainright.com

CHAPTER 11

RACE YOUR PLAN ON RACE DAY

"It does not matter how slowly you go
as long as you do not stop."

—*CONFUCIUS*

FOR EVERY MAJOR EVENT OR RACE I'VE DONE, INCLUDING
my mastectomy surgery, I created a race plan. I did this for my
early sprint triathlons, Olympic distance triathlons, the mara-
thon, the half marathons, the Half Ironman, and every single
100-mile bike ride I've done (which at this point, I've lost count
of how many that has been). I do love a long bike ride.

A race plan is a guide you follow when you are pushing
your body and mind to do something that's out of your com-
fort zone. It grounds you and holds you steady as you proceed
toward your goal. Many coaches have told their athletes, me
included, "Create your race plan, and then race your plan."

Athletes who take themselves seriously prepare. Multisport
athletes in particular prepare. For those of us with chronic
health conditions, we have to plan everyday life. When we
become athletes, the chronic health condition blends into our
race preparation. For a recent half marathon I did, I wrote a
detailed plan that started a full week before race day. The reason

I start so early is that I want to get myself into the mindset of what is to come. I want to be sure that I'm keeping my blood sugar in an ideal range, since any bad low blood sugars depletes my glycogen, or sugar stores in my liver and muscles, which I will need on race day. I also want to be certain that my body is well hydrated, which means I plan out and keep track of how many glasses of water or herbal tea or Nuun-tablet-filled-water I'm drinking every day for a week.

I also look at the work stress in my life leading up to the event. My goal is to minimize my stress, and minimize surprises that could and likely would derail my focus going into the race. This helps me sleep at least 8 or 9 hours every night before race day. I love having a race plan. I love making my athletic events as celebratory as possible and having a detailed race plan elevates the event to rock star status. After all, you and I are worth it. Take a moment to read the following components of a race plan, then begin to write one for your event.

FIVE COMPONENTS OF A RACE PLAN

These five components of a race plan intertwine, overlap, and weave together. The harder I push myself physically in an athletic event, the fuzzier my thinking can get. This is due primarily to the intensity of the physical push, so having my plan written down makes a positive difference in my ability to manage diabetes or other health decisions. Reviewing the Race Plan in the days, hours, and even minutes before the race begins helps my brain keep track of what I am doing, and need to continue to do, as the race progresses.

Look at these five components as a whole and then craft each section for yourself. I also give you several examples of race plans that you can modify to make your own.

Component 1. Mindset

How will you mentally approach your race? What stories will you tell yourself as the event approaches and you do the event? What mantras will you say to yourself as you push your body? The two subcomponents for this part of the plan are Meditation/Deep Breathing and Mantras for the race.

Component 2. Pre-Race

I outline what I will eat, how much I will sleep, and what stress, in as much as I can control it, I will allow in my life for two or three days before the event. I like to be specific about what I will do the week, and a few days, before the race. I make sure I plan to arrive at the race venue well in advance of the scheduled start time. In the case of a triathlon, I want to make sure I have time to set up my transition area, to walk the transition routes, to get my body marked, to go to the bathroom at least once (often more times), and to have time to do any scheduled warm-ups, all with calm and focus. For most events, I plan to arrive at least an hour in advance.

Additionally, if I can, I drive or ride or walk the race route in advance, so that I know the course. One year, I did a new-to-me sprint distance triathlon in a suburb far from my house. I recruited my biking friend Tammy to ride the bike route with me. I arrived early to the transition site and I walked the area, familiarizing myself with the lake, and the area surrounding where the transition area was mapped to be. (I got all that from the triathlon website.) When Tammy arrived, we discussed the parking situation (being adjacent to a residential neighborhood might be tricky on race morning). I had read the Athletes Handbook that the race provided, which had given me a warning about the parking situation. Knowing what you need to do before the event you're doing and having a clear plan for all activities (like parking) before event day is smart to do for every race or athletic event you do.

Then Tammy and I got our bikes ready for our practice ride; we made sure our tires were pumped up and the brakes were working and we had all our nutrition and hydration ready to go. Off we went. I had printed out a map of the route, and we followed the race biking route exactly. We rode the route at a very leisurely pace and we laughed and told stories the entire 15-mile route. We even made up names for ourselves, along with old-school very proper accents. That made us laugh even harder. My name was Agnes and Tammy was Abigail. Our backstory was that both of us had divorced wealthy husbands who had given us huge settlements, allowing us to purchase several yachts that we saw on the lake as we rode past. The triathlon was the next week, and as I rode the course at twice the pace Abigail and Agnes had ridden it, I remembered our laughter and silly stories. That gave me energy to ride my bike even faster.

Another thing I make sure to have in the Pre-Race section of my race plan is to practice my transition flow one more time the week of a triathlon. I have the entire thing written down on index cards that are clipped together for easy access, and easy reviewing. I practice the transitions mentally and physically. I've learned over the years that kinesthetically practicing the order I will take off my bike shoes, put on my run shoes, put on my sunglasses and my bike helmet, take off my bike helmet, and put on my sun visor helps me remember the order when I'm doing it at lightning speed in the transition area. Remember, the length of time you take in transition does count toward your total race time. The more you practice, the faster and smoother it will go.

There are many parts to the Pre-Race component of the race plan. Taking time to write it down, to review it, and to practice it are vital to success. The eight subcomponents I outline for myself in this Pre-Race section of the race plan are sleep, nutrition, hydration, work plan, training, therapies, diabetes management, and day before the race.

Component 3. Gear

Early on, a coach told me to never use new gear at a race. I didn't understand why this was until I wore a new pair of swim goggles in a race. It was awful; I didn't have them adjusted to my face and head, and they kept falling off. Luckily, it was a sprint distance triathlon, and the swim was over fairly quickly; nonetheless, my eyes hurt for the rest of the race. If you want new gear for a big event or race, make sure you've owned the item for at least a week and tried the gear out for at least one or two exercise sessions. That way the gear won't be brand new and untested.

In my race plan, I make sure that two days before the event I have gathered all the gear I will wear and use, and I make sure everything is clean and ready to go.

In addition to the athletic gear, I additionally have a diabetes gear plan. Whatever your health challenge, knowing what you need during your event and having that plan written down will be a big help.

For example, I like to wear an additional pump set, in the event my primary set falls off because I pull it off accidentally or it sweats off. I also make sure for longer bike ride events to have a needle and spare half-filled bottle of insulin along in the off chance I have an insulin pump failure. I often carry a small blood testing kit with me on bike rides, in addition to having my continuous glucose monitor. Having a plan B for my essential diabetes gear provides great relief and calm as I mentally prepare for my event.

Component 4. Day of the Race

I outline as exactly as possible what I will eat, drink, and think as the race progresses and also what I will be doing with my gear. There are a number of components I like to write down and consider related to the day of the event I've trained for many weeks to complete. Here they are outlined for you. You will notice, the Pre-Race and Day-of-Event components of my race plan are nearly always the longest parts.

Race-Specific Rules & Goals for the Race

For this part of my race plan, I make sure I take a moment to review any race-specific rules. USAT, the governing body of USA Triathlon, has very specific rules for USAT-sanctioned races. For example, no matter what, you cannot and should not draft on the bike. Meaning you need to stay three bike lengths behind the cyclist in front of you. The other USAT rule that is different from running races is you cannot listen to music for any part of the race. Meaning you can't have earbuds or headphones in your ears on the bike or for the run.

I don't put this next part in my race plan, but while I am racing, I make sure I'm following all the regular rules of the road, especially if any part of the race is on public roads. Most races have lots of volunteers on the route guiding the athletes on the turns to be sure everyone stays as safe as possible. I do remind myself to pay attention to these generous volunteers and say thank you to them as I'm racing by.

In this part of my race plan, I also include any goals I have for the race/event. For example, if I have a time goal for the race or if I have something related to how I want to feel as I'm racing. It helps to write your goals down and have them visible in front of you, because this will help you discover if you have any secret goals. Secret goals are often unrealistic, hopeful goals that you hide from yourself and for sure from others. The problem with having secret goals is that if or when you don't achieve them, a profound sense of letdown and disappointment can permeate all the amazing things you did accomplish. Thus, make an effort to get clear with yourself about your goals for your event/race, and then include them in your race plan.

Pacing Plan

When you're doing a long endurance event, knowing how fast you want to go at various points during the race will help you keep track of how you're doing. For example, in longer bike events, such as 100-mile bike rides, I like to finish in under 7 or 8 hours. That means that I need to keep a steady pace of at least 15 miles per hour. When I start the event, I like to give myself the first hour to keep a pace of 12 to 13 miles per hour. Then as my body is warmed up and I'm in the groove of the ride, I like to up my pace to 15 to 16 miles per hour. I've always studied the route we will be on, to become familiar with the elevation and any other challenges that might present themselves. This helps me plan my pacing.

As you gain confidence and experience racing and doing endurance events, taking some time to plan your pacing will help you achieve the goals you've laid out for yourself. I find it also helps me get motivated during my training days.

Nutrition

It's critical to be clear about your nutrition plan in longer endurance events. This is especially true if you have diabetes, or any other health challenge that relates to your eating plan. It's important to not consume products you haven't practiced with and trained your digestive system to understand. I like to write down exactly what I will eat and when I will eat it. There's an adage that many endurance athletes use, and you've likely heard it: "Drink before you get thirsty and eat before you get hungry." The race rationale to this adage is that it takes hormones to warn you that you're thirsty or hungry, and if your body needs to send your brain messages with hormones, your body isn't using all your energy on racing.

As much as I can the day before and the morning before a race, I make a concerted effort to eat home-cooked food that I know 100 percent what's in it. I did a half marathon in Duluth, Minnesota, and five of us drove up the day before the race. We purposely rented an apartment at the University of Minnesota Duluth that had a kitchen. This allowed us to eat the food we prepared and brought with us. Too many athlete friends have made the mistake of eating out the day before a big race and gotten food poisoning or disrupted their digestive system. I do my best to avoid that happening.

The other thing I've learned over time to do on race day is to get up three hours before the race start to eat a quick breakfast. Three hours allows my digestive system time to fully digest the food I eat for breakfast. It also allows my "insulin on board" (the insulin I took to cover the carbohydrates I ate for breakfast) to be mostly out of my system. This is an effective early morning nutrition strategy for athletes with insulin-dependent diabetes. Turns out, all my professional endurance athlete friends tell me this is a strategy they use before a big race. Giving the body time to digest and clear food out helps the body be fueled up and focused on the race.

Hydration

Being well hydrated before, during, and after any significant athletic event is essential for athletic success. Water regulates body temperature, and it lubricates your joints. It helps transport nutrients to give you energy as you are moving. In short, your body can't perform at its highest level if you aren't well hydrated. Mid-race you might notice you feel tired, you might get muscle cramps, become dizzy, or other unfavorable consequences.

How much water you in particular should drink depends on you and what you've learned about your hydration needs. One of my run coaches suggested that ideally each of us drinks half our body weight in ounces each day. Specifically drinking water. I weigh a little less than 160 pounds, so that would be 80 ounces of water a day. For me, my goal is to drink 10 cups of water or water similar beverages a day. I like herbal teas and that counts as water.

The following is a guideline from the American Council on Exercise on how much water to consume before, during, and after exercise.

- 17–20 ounces of water 2–3 hours prior to exercise

- 8 ounces of water 20–30 minutes before exercise or during your warm-up
- 7–10 ounces of water every 10–20 minutes during exercise
- 8 ounces of water within 30 minutes after exercise[1]

It's important for athletes, especially during preseason workouts, to measure how much fluid you lose in each session to get a good indication of how much water replacement you actually need. This is done easily by stepping on a scale before and after each workout, noting the amount of weight loss. It is recommended that athletes drink 16–24 ounces of water for every pound lost during activity. It is very important to replace fluid lost during activity. Not replacing water may lead to dehydration. If an athlete is participating in a high-intensity activity for a prolonged period of time (more than an hour), replacing fluid loss with a sports drink is helpful as it also replenishes electrolytes. Just remember to steer clear of sports drinks containing high levels of sugar. I've done the weighing before and after long workout sessions a few times, and learning how much weight I've lost is fascinating. In essence, what I keep learning is "drink more water."

Speaking of sports drinks, be sure to find out what sports drinks your event or race is going to offer and be sure you practice with that exact sports drink. Again, you want to be sure you've trained your body to perform well with anything you plan to put in it on race day.

One more detail about hydration I want to mention: what to do about peeing if you're drinking all these liquids? I confess, I think about details like this quite a bit. Turns out, chances are you are going to sweat most of it out of your body.

It surprises me time and time again how rarely I need to pee when going for a six-to-eight-hour bike ride or a three-to-four-hour run (yes, it's true, I'm not fast so I'm out there moving my body for long training sessions). That said, when I was training for the Half Ironman back in 2009, upon the advice of the coaches, I did train myself to pee while riding my bike. Meaning I simply started peeing, right through my triathlon shorts. The bummer was that the pee would run down my leg and sometimes get into my bike shoes and socks. I had to plan these peeing extravaganzas for times I had plain water in one of my water bottles to rinse off my legs, socks, and shoes. I did all of that while still riding my bike at a good clip. I did not enjoy these peeing excursions. Plus, I had to wash my bike shoes when I got home so they wouldn't start to smell. Ironman events these days have lots of porta-potties on the bike and run routes, so random peeing is not necessary. This is true for many organized bike and run events and races. In general, if you use the porta-potties before the event starts, chances are good you won't need to pee until the race or event is finished.

Race Day Health Strategies

For those of us with a health challenge, putting reminders of what you want to do during the event/race will help you remember and take action accordingly. As a person with type 1 diabetes, the big things I make sure I've thought about and taken action on are

- Do I have enough insulin in my pump?
- Is my spare set inserted so if something happens to the main set, I have a backup?

- Is my continuous glucose monitor in a good place on my body and does it have enough tape and SkinTac on it so it won't fall off?
- Do I have enough quick-acting sugars with me, in case of low blood sugar?

Take some time to think through your particular health strategies that you want to have in place for your event. Slow down, breathe deeply, and consider what you need and want. Then make it happen.

To recap, the five subcomponents of this Day-of-the-Race component that I outline in my race plan include my goals for the race, my pacing plan, nutrition, hydration, and diabetes strategies. Take some time to think about and design your Day-of-the-Race plan. This will help the whole thing come alive!

Component 5: Post-Race

Written down, a post-race plan helps me transition from the race itself back to the rest of my life. It's easy to forget to eat or drink once the event is accomplished. One of the key things I often forget immediately after an event is to take insulin for the post-race meal I eat. As you can imagine, forgetting this insulin results in skyrocketing blood sugar, which sucks. I hate the feeling of super high blood sugar, especially when it is avoidable. The secret is to remember to take insulin as I'm eating that post-race meal. The other thing I've noticed post-race is that if I've done an anaerobic push at the end of a big event, that anaerobic surge will cause my body to need more insulin, and I can have a post-event really high blood sugar. I've learned over time to not fully bolus insulin to cover this particular high blood sugar as within an hour or so, my blood sugar will come down on its own.

The key is to learn *your* body, and what you need for yourself to have the most successful event possible. Take a moment and think about your health challenges. What do you need at the end of your event to finish as successfully as possible? All that training you did gave you lots of excellent guidance about what you and your body need. Be sure to keep listening to your body. It is very wise.

One more thing I put into the Post-Race component of my race plan is how I want to spend time after the event. I talked at length about this aspect in chapter 6, and this component of your race plan might not need critical attention, but for those who tend to operate alone in the world, like I do, having this in your post-race plan will help you remember that you are connected, that you have community, and that you belong. I often forget this, so I consider this an important item for my race plan. I ask myself this question: "Who do you want with you at and after the event?"

This affects how much social media you use leading up to the big day and after the event. Social media can be very supportive and encouraging. It can also undermine confidence. Accomplishing a big goal takes a lot of energy and focus; I do best by having only positive people around.

One year I trained for a 100-mile bike ride essentially by myself, and I realized that I wanted people at the end of the ride to celebrate with me. I invited three work colleagues to come. They all said yes and, as I crossed the finish line and saw them there, cheering me, my eyes filled with tears of happiness and connection. It meant the world to see them and hug them, and it wrapped up the ride in a bow of joy!

RACE PLAN EXAMPLES

Here are three sample race plans from races I've done in the past. Please consider them as general guides. The first is for a half marathon I did not too long ago. Second is for a duathlon (run/bike/run) I did. The third one is for a 100-mile bike ride. The first example follows the guidelines I outlined here. The second and third examples are earlier race plans, and they show how I got better and better at writing them.

I didn't just write these plans out of thin air; the ratios and guidelines listed in the plans are specific to my body, my level of fitness, and my experience during training sessions. As you craft your race plan, it will be custom to you and what you need.

My best guidance is to have fun with it. Doing your athletic event is taking charge of your health and your life. Enjoy the process!

RACE PLAN EXAMPLE ONE: HALF MARATHON IN DULUTH, MINNESOTA

Component 1. Mindset

Meditation and Deep Breathing

All this week, I will meditate for at least 30 minutes right when I wake up each morning. This will help me keep my stress and anxiety in check. I am wearing a hair tie around my wrist and anytime I notice tension rising in my body, I will snap the hair tie. This is a reminder to breathe deeply and relax. My goal is to relax and enjoy all the work that I've done to get me here.

Mantras for the Race

- I am strong.
- Smile, I love running.
- Believe in this body. This body is strong. This body is capable.
- Feel the strength in this body. This is mine. I've done the work. Own it.
- Notice the trees. Notice the people. I belong.

Component 2. Pre-Race

Sleep

I will be in bed by 8:30 p.m. every night this week. All electronics are off by 8:30 p.m. and asleep by 9:00 p.m. My goal is to get at least 8 hours of sleep every night, maybe even 9 hours.

Nutrition

This is a week of super-clean eating. No gluten. Not one drop. No meat (this one isn't difficult!). Minimal dairy (I do eat some cheese, but I'm cutting way back this week). Make sure I'm getting enough calories and not overeating. It's all about balance.

As I typically do, I cooked on Sunday. My recipes this week are Atakilt Wat (an Ethiopian vegetable stew with cabbage, potato, and carrots) with added tofu and then quinoa chickpea salad with dill dressing. For breakfast, I will have my regular chia pudding, which is nutritious and delicious with fresh berries. Thrown in for fun and extra veggies, I will have a few salad jars.

Hydration

The weather in Duluth for race morning, June 18, looks pretty spectacular. That said, I tend to suffer when it's extra humid and hot. To be as ready as possible, I will make sure to drink enough water and electrolytes every day this week. Nuun tablets are my friend.

Work Plan

This week my work duties are light. I arranged my schedule so this would be the case. Minimal meetings. Minimal grading. Low stress. I'm taking both Thursday and Friday off. Thursday so I can focus on packing and mental prep. Friday so we can drive up to Duluth.

Training

I'm cutting out all weight lifting. I will do a bit of core work and some stretching. No barbells or kettlebells this week. I will run 4 miles on Tuesday and 2 miles on Friday morning before heading to Duluth. No swimming this week. I will do a bit of biking, about 12 miles, commuting to and from a work celebration. And that's it. Reminding myself that tapering *is* a good idea!

Therapies

Getting my body 100 percent in race mode is my goal. It might be a bit of overkill, but I'm willing to give it a try. On Monday, I have an acupuncture session with my incredible acupuncturist John Falls. On Tuesday, I'm going in for a chiropractic session. Dr. Sadie helps my hips and neck be in alignment. On Wednesday, I will see my massage therapist. Sarah gets my feet, my calves, and my quads ready for the race.

Diabetes

I make sure I had on a fresh continuous glucose monitor that is securely attached with a Type One Style sticker. Additionally, I put on a new insulin pump set on Thursday mid-day. That way, at 6:00 a.m. when I start the race, I will have a good set working with plenty of insulin. To make 100 percent sure that I have my diabetes bases covered, on Friday I will put on an additional set. (In case the one that's attached to the pump accidentally pulls or sweats off, I have a backup set ready to go.)

Also related to diabetes, I will do my very best to keep my "time-in-range" at 80–85% for the whole week. That means keeping my blood sugar between 70 mg/dl and 180 mg/dl. With the goal of not having *any* low blood sugars on Thursday or Friday before the Saturday race. That way my liver and my muscles will be glycogen-ready and topped off.

Day before the Race

I will get up at 5:00 a.m. to meditate. Then I eat my chia pudding breakfast. Sam, my dog, and I will head out for a quick, easy, slow two-mile run. Quick shower and put my already packed suitcase and cooler with food for the day in the car. By 8:45 a.m. I will be headed to pick up Nadine. I've got our lodging info printed out. We will meet up with Jenny and Brooke in Duluth.

Once we get settled at the University of Minnesota Duluth apartment where we will sleep for two nights, we will head to the Race Expo and survey the area. Jenny and Brooke are both spectating, so we'll make plans for meeting up.

Both Nadine and I will have our lunch and dinner items with us for the day before the race. After all, eating out means unknown preparation and ingredients. My goal is to keep my blood sugar above 90 mg/dl all day. And of course below 180 mg/dl. That requires that I know exactly what I'm putting in my body.

Last, I will get my drop bag ready for after the race, and then of course, to bed early!

Component 3. Gear

Run Gear

I am a bit obsessed with lists. Nothing like a good list to feel a sense of control and readiness.

Here's my run gear list for this half marathon. Remember, Duluth weather can be very unpredictable. Very cold to very hot. It could pour rain. Gotta be ready with all the options.

- Ear warmer
- Poncho
- Body glide for underarms
- Neck cooling options
- Run gloves
- Visor and hat
- Socks & shoes
- Run bra & run underwear
- Shorts—Senita flower shorts
- Tank—Run Minnesota
- T-shirt—long sleeve from Women Run The Cities
- Blue compression sleeves for calves
- Pink jacket
- Neck gaiter
- Flipbelt waist band
- Nutrition: UCAN, gels, sport jelly beans, Smarties

- Water bottle, the side one to wear
- Nuun tabs
- Bug spray
- Sunscreen
- Clothes for after bag: sandals, socks, another rain poncho, hat, ear warmer, another shirt, another pair of shorts, leggings, wash cloth in a baggie, wipes of some kind, face mask, snacks, another pump set, phone charger option
- Warm items I can wear early and then toss aside before starting: sweatshirt, neck gaiter, sweat pants.

Diabetes Gear

- I like to have a clear diabetes list too. As I mentioned above, I will put on a fresh pump set on Thursday, two days before the race.
- I will put on an extra pump set on Friday in the event my primary set falls off because I pull it off accidentally or it sweats off.
- The Dexcom G6 continuous glucose monitor I wear lasts for 10 days. I put on a new CGM on Monday, so race day will be day 5 of a 10-day set.

Component 4. Day of the Race

The half marathon race starts at 6:00 a.m. All of us runners *must* take the bus to the race start. The bus from UMD where my friends and I are sleeping Friday and Saturday nights leaves UMD at 4:30 a.m. Nadine and I will get up a bit before 4:00 a.m. I will do a 5-minute meditation. I will have all my clothes and food laid out ready to put on quickly and grab to leave. I will boil water to make my chia pudding that I will carry with me and eat on the bus. I will have a plastic spoon and the chia pudding is in a small plastic recyclable container.

As we board the bus, we hand off our after bags. Any warm clothing we have on we can drop at the race start. Goodwill will pick up all that we drop.

Race Goals

- Have negative splits
- Walk fast for 30 seconds every mile
- Finish the race in 2 hours and 40–45 minutes (that's an average pace of 12:30)
- Smile and have fun
- Feel relaxed, calm, and joyful

Pacing

- Miles 1, 2, 3: 13-minute miles
- Miles 4, 5, 6: 12:45-minute miles
- Miles 7, 8: 12:30-minute miles
- Miles 9, 10, 11: 12-minute miles
- Mile 12 to the end: 11:30-minute miles

Nutrition

- I will eat my chia pudding breakfast on the bus to the start of the race. I will take no insulin for this 450 calorie/30 grams of carbohydrate meal. This will be about 1 hour before the race starts. I've practiced this eating strategy and it works for me.
- At 5:30 a.m., 30 minutes before the race starts, I will eat a UCAN packet.

- I will carry with me 4 gel packets, 2 Sport Bean packets, 1 UCAN packet, and at least 8 rolls of Smarties. These will be in my FlipBelt Adjustable Run Belt.
- My plan is to track my blood sugar as I run. At mile 6 I will eat the second UCAN.
- I will eat a gel/Sport Beans at mile 3, mile 9, and maybe mile 11.
- In case of low blood sugars, I will eat a 6-gram carbohydrate Smartie.

Hydration

- I will have my 10-ounce FlipBelt curved water bottle that fits easily in the side pocket of my Senita running shorts. I will drink a glass of water with a Nuun tablet (for electrolytes) right when I wake up at 4:00 a.m.
- I will drink the full 10 ounces of water while I'm riding the bus. I will refill the bottle before we start the run. I will use the porta-potty at least once.
- As I'm running, I know that there will be official water stations at miles 2, 4, 6, 7, 8, 9, 10, 11, and 12. As my water bottle gets empty, I will refill at the water stations. I have a rhythm of drinking water at least every mile. In my FlipBelt, I will carry a few Nuun tabs in case of heat and humidity.

Diabetes

- I will study my CGM tracing from the day and night before, and I will study how much insulin my pump gave me through the night as I slept. In prep for breakfast, I will take this into consideration.

- Since the race starts at 6:00 a.m., I will turn off the SLEEP pattern on my pump at 4:45 a.m. and at 5:00 a.m. I will turn on the ACTIVITY setting.

Component 5: Post-Race

After the race, I will find Jenny, Brooke, and Nadine and celebrate my accomplishment and hear about Nadine's accomplishments, since she is superfast. I will ask Jenny and Brooke how the spectating went.

I will find my After Bag and make sure I'm warm and fully covered in sunscreen and bug spray.

I will need to keep close track of my blood sugar. I tend to spike after a strong athletic effort, so I've got to turn off the ACTIVITY setting and give myself an insulin bolus as soon as I finish the race.

We will find our way to the Run Minnesota gathering spot and hang out and watch the marathoners finish their race! It will be *so fun* to celebrate with my incredible Run Minnesota teammates. I'm especially excited to see Tanya P, Tanya L, Linda, and Kathryn cross the finish line. Maybe I will even get to see Coach Danny cross the finish line. He's going to run this marathon extra fast!

We will find a delicious lunch and then later we will meet up for dinner with the Run Minnesota group.

Once we get back to our UMD apartment that shower will feel fabulous! As will getting into bed for a delicious sleep.

RACE PLAN EXAMPLE TWO: OAKDALE DUATHLON

Goals: Finish smiling and feeling strong
Mantra: *This* is living life!

Two Days before Race:

- Make sure my continuous glucose monitor is inserted in a good location and has enough adhesive on and around it.
- Go for 30-minute easy run.
- Keep blood glucose level higher than 70 ml/dl at all times (to keep glycogen topped off in my liver).
- Make sure I have directions to race venue and make sure I have a plan for parking my car and walking with my bike to the venue.
- Get clothing ready and packed.
- Check bike (tires, brakes, derailleur, chain); make sure everything is clean and oiled.
- Check over my run shoes. Make sure the laces are set exactly how I want them.
- Go to sleep by 10:00 p.m. so I get 8–9 hours of sleep each night.

Day before Race:

- Make sure CGM is on and working
- Make sure pump insulin is fresh and working, put on an extra set as backup
- Keep blood glucose over 70 mg/dl at all times
- Eat very healthy; all meals are known foods and carb counts

- Prep breakfast food for race day
- Pack clothes and gear
- Have index card reminders of mantras & plans ready to go
- Check bike; go for easy 30-minute spin
- Go for easy 15-minute run
- Go to sleep by 9:00 p.m.

Race Day!

5:00 a.m.—wake up and test blood sugar. If in normal range, take 100% bolus for breakfast food:

- 3 eggs scrambled with spinach
- 3 corn tortillas = 20 grams carbs
- 1 grapefruit (whole) = 27 grams carbs
- ½ c soy milk with tea = 5 grams carbs
- 1 tsp honey in tea = 6 grams carbs
  - » Total carbs for breakfast: 58g

Feed dog; take him on quick walk

Get dressed, wearing warm clothes over race clothes

Bring or affix race number

Remember water bottles*

*Total water bottles: FOUR—two for bike (one with Skratch Lab [45 g carbs] and one with plain water with Nuun electrolyte tabs), another for the first run, and a small one for the second run.

15-minute sitting meditation focusing on breathing and relaxing

Prepare recovery shake for after race

Put bike, gear bag, and cooler in car

6:45 a.m.—Depart for race venue; play dance-happy music in the car.

7:15 a.m.—Arrive at the race venue. (The transition area opens at 7:30 a.m.)

7:30 a.m.—Turn BASAL rate down on insulin pump to 75 percent for three and a half hours.

Sign in: Get race number, find transition area, set up transition, go to bathroom, check blood sugar, apply sunscreen, mentally review nutrition and hydration strategies. Make sure to have testers and glucose tabs in all places.

Gear review: Take bike cleat covers off my bike shoes so I can put them on with ease in the transition area after the swim. Make sure bike shoes are ready to go.

Mental strategy: Review race strategy. Breathe. Smile lots. Keep it light, keep it positive. Relax. Remind myself this is for *fun*!

Mantra: This is fun! I am happy. This is what happy and fun feel like.

Race prep: Jump around a bit to get and stay warm. Remember being cold is OK! Leave base camp cold!
　Check blood sugar (BG) while waiting at race start:

- If BG is below 100, eat half banana
- If BG is 100 to 200—maybe eat half a banana

- If BG is 200 to 250—no action
- If BG is above 250—mini bolus, *no more than* 1 unit. Really check in about this

9:00 a.m.—Race starts! *Run* **three miles**. Average 12- to 13-minute miles. Take it easy. OK if at the back of the pack. Total time will be 40 minutes.

At end of run, while moving, test BG:

- If BG below 90, eat 2–3 glucose tabs.
- If BG between 90 and 200, wait until on the bike and then start with Skratch Lab, drink entire bottle (45 grams carbs).
- If BG over 200, drink more water, notice if trending up or down, if up, consider very mini bolus.

At the end of the bike, look at CGM and consider eating gel packet, especially if under 130 mg/dl.

9:40 a.m. T1 (First Transition)— Change out of run shoes, take off fuel belt, put on helmet, put on bike shoes.

9:43 a.m. Bike Out—14-mile bike
- Do bike in just over an hour. Ride with focus and power. This is so *fun*! My favorite part.

10:50 a.m. Bike In, T2 (Second Transition)
- Dismount, helmet off, switch shoes, put on fuel belt as moving toward Run Out. Test BG as walking to Run Out.

10:53 a.m. Run Out—2.5 mile run
- If BG below 90, eat a few glucose tabs.
- If BG between 90 and 200—consider eating gel that is in the run belt pocket.
- If BG over 200, drink more water, notice if trending up or down, if up, consider very mini bolus *and* stop temp basal rate.

Mental strategy: The first quarter-mile run will hurt; it always does. Keep moving and breathe into it. Focus on my body and send my legs love and strength. It will and it *always* does shift and ease up.

Last mile: Consider pushing at this point. See if I can do a 10-minute mile pace down the home stretch.

Post-race: Race should be done for me by 11:15 a.m. Smile! Celebrate! I did it! First multisport race since October 2009 is in the bag! Pack up gear. Snap photos.

Recovery: Almond milk with protein powder: yum! Eat a healthy post-race recovery meal. Watch BGs for the rest of the day. Warm shower. Celebration lunch with friends! Go to bed early.

RACE PLAN EXAMPLE THREE: AMERICAN DIABETES ASSOCIATION TOUR DE CURE IN IOWA: 100-MILE BIKE RIDE

Mantras: I am strong. I can do this. I ride for my dog Riley. I ride for myself. I ride for all who have diabetes.

Day before Ride:

- Fill water bottles
- Double check everything on bike: chain, brakes, tires
- Pin ride number on jersey
- Lay out bike clothes, helmet, gloves, shoes, sunglasses
- Get nutrition ready: Skratch Lab drink mix in baggies, make PB&J with gluten-free bread
- Put on extra infusion set for insulin pump
- Charge phone battery; bring extra battery
- Make sure have enough test strips & glucose tabs
- Make sure have a needle and bottle of insulin in my seat bag, just in case
- Visualize success, keeping a 14- to 16-mph pace, breathing well
- All day, make sure blood glucose stays above 70.
- In bed by 9:00 p.m.

Day of Ride

4:15 a.m.—Wake up, take insulin for breakfast 45 grams of carbs, but only take insulin for 30 grams. Take 3 units. Eat oatmeal, walnuts, berries, almond milk, two eggs, tea, apple

4:30 a.m.—Turn down basal rate to -20 percent for 8 hours

4:45 a.m.—Pack
- Bike
- Clothes and flip flops in backpack
- Food and water
- Check tools in back pouch
- Bring phone charger
- Apply sunscreen

5:00 a.m.—Depart hotel

5:10 a.m.—Arrive at ride start; find place to store backpack ***Check BG—bring extra juice. Drink if I need it. Calibrate Dexcom CGM

6:00 a.m.—Ride start

Every hour: eat 45 to 50 grams of carbs: Gels & Skratch
- Test blood sugar at every rest stop, make sure CGM is matching finger blood tests. If needed, do micro-boluses (1 unit or less at a time)

Post Event/Recovery

- Hang out with fun people and enjoy this major accomplishment!
- Be sure to watch blood sugars with care. Take insulin for post-recovery food.
- Drive home with happy music playing

There you have it. Three example race plans. You can see that they are different based on my experience writing them and my experience as an athlete. Be kind and gentle with yourself as you craft your race plan. There are many ways to create a race plan. As you keep doing events and noticing your success, your race plans will evolve too. Try out the five components I offer you, and make them work for you and your event.

TRY THIS

Journal

For one of your upcoming races/events, sketch out a race plan for yourself. Which of the race plan components call out to you? Write these down. A race plan can be a work in progress.

Consider sharing your race plan with the people you trained with. I love sharing my race plan with my community and seeing their race plans. Getting new ideas and reassurance helps with race confidence!

Notes

1. "How Hydration Affects Performance," Evolution Nutrition, ACE Insights, April 29, 2015, https://www.acefitness.org/resources/pros/expert-articles/5397/how-hydration-affects-performance/

Resources

Ways Meditation Changes the Brain: https://www.forbes.com/sites/alicegwalton/2015/02/09/7-ways-meditation-can-actually-change-the-brain/#346bc9b41465

CHAPTER 12

OVER THE LONG HAUL

"Love yourself, for who and what you
are; protect your dream and develop
your talent to the fullest extent."

—*JOAN BENOIT SAMUELSON*

YOUR RACE IS OVER.

How do you feel? Along with happiness and a feeling of accomplishment can come feelings of letdown, loss, and bewilderment about what to do next, which are entirely normal after your big event is over. When I trained for and accomplished with flying colors that 400-mile bike ride across Colorado, I was shocked at how lost and sad I felt when it was over. My energy had been 100 percent devoted to preparing for and doing the ride. I cried most of the way home, and I kept crying as I carried my gear into my house. I was overjoyed that I had accomplished the event, but now I was completely lost. I had no idea what to do or what to focus on next.

The next day, I called Coach Nicole and asked her what athletes did after accomplishing a big goal. She told me it was important to feel it all: happy about the accomplishment and sad for it being over. She encouraged me to do a few celebratory things, like getting a massage and going out for drinks and staying out late. And after a few days, start looking for another event I could do. This was before I'd discovered triathlon, so I wasn't sure what that might be, but I realized I would find another challenge and that alone was reassuring.

This chapter explores two things. One is how you continue to be an endurance athlete over the years. The other is how to be an endurance athlete as you age. Both are connected to the idea of the long haul. Being an endurance athlete year after year, as we age, requires figuring out how to hang in there.

Over the years, I found a lot more athletic events to do. At the end of each one, I feel a mix of big happiness and big sadness. I understand now that both are normal. At this point, I've been an endurance athlete for more than twenty years. I understand the ebb and flow of the season of training and resting.

I train differently during the various months of the year. Meaning, in November, December, and January, I focus on building my strength and maintaining my fitness. I don't attempt to do nine workouts a week (which I do when I'm training for an Olympic distance or a longer distance triathlon). I also don't try to ride my bike for 10 to 15 hours a week, which is what I do when I am training for a 100-mile bike ride. Since I live in Minnesota (with cold and snowy winter months), I add in cross country skiing, which to me feels like dancing as I glide along the surface of the snow. I am grateful that endurance athletic events still engage my heart, soul, and body.

This isn't true for everyone. A few of my friends who worked out with me in my early days no longer participate in endurance sports; they've found other activities. One became a disc jockey. Another is an expert knitter. Someone else got into recreational volleyball. On the other end of the spectrum, a few of them have done full Ironman events (2.4-mile swim, 112-mile bike, 26.2-mile run) with regularity and great enthusiasm. One woman does extreme endurance cycling events where she rides longer than 200 miles in one stretch.

What matters is that each of us found our way. Trying out endurance athletics is one powerful way to regain your health, get you back in your body. You may discover that continuing to be an endurance athlete isn't for you. Perhaps it served you in getting back into regular exercise and movement of some sort. Maybe it helped you remember that you can have a good relationship with food. In any case, whether you continue being an endurance athlete or not, giving it a try is worth it. You will discover more about yourself!

RECORD THE EXPERIENCE

When your event is over, it's the cycle of life. You get to decide what you'll do next. Reflection on accomplishments is a beautiful thing to do at the completion of a major athletic race/event. I reflect on what I liked about the event, what went well, how my body responded to all the training and how it did during the race or event. Often, I write a detailed race report that I publish on my blog. I recount my emotions and my blood sugars. I think about how hard I did, or did not, push myself. I reflect about how much anxiety and excitement I navigated before and during the race or event.

By doing this, I can review my Race Report when I'm lining up my next athletic goals. I also spend some time feeling all the emotions of the accomplishment. I like describing the depth of emotions I feel before, during, and after an event. In my case, I feel many emotions. Maybe it's because I am fully present in my body for the entire race, and emotions are felt in the body.

My awareness of my emotions is heightened because these days I am tuned into my body. Taking a moment to write down both the physical and emotional experience reminds me to bring this awareness to my daily life. I encourage you to do the same. Having a log of how your races/events went is helpful to have going forward.

ONE WAY

I am happy to report that, despite or maybe in spite of everything I have survived, I enjoy my life. I'm aging, and athletic things often get harder as we age. We tend to get slower as we age. That said, I have so many amazing role models who are ten to twenty-plus years older than me. These older people show me that aging needn't be something to dread. One of the secrets to aging successfully is to keep moving.

These days, I run year-round at the local high school track with a group from the Minneapolis YWCA. Laurie, the coach, creates interval workouts for us to do each week. We run outside as long as there isn't snow on the ground. Once snow accumulates, we go inside to the indoor track. They don't plow the outdoor track. Too bad, because it feels safer to be outside with all the COVID variants and versions of the flu going around.

These interval track workouts have helped me get incrementally faster at running. I did a 10K (6.2 miles) with my writing friend Shirlene in 2019. It was the Monster Dash. That race took me 1 hour and 22 minutes to complete. In 2021, I did the same route and same race again. Due to all the interval training and weightlifting I had been doing, I did the Monster Dash eight minutes faster than two years earlier. I was two years older and I was 8 minutes faster. That result caused me to do a happy dance of joy. Turns out, it is possible to get faster as you age. What matters is consistency and paying attention.

In June of 2021, upon the advice and ongoing coaching of Dana Roseman (MPH, CDCES, RDN, a Certified Diabetes Educator, and a Registered Dietitian who works with Diabetes Integrated Services), I began taking Ozempic, and I started doing full-body weightlifting twice a week for an hour. Ozempic is a semaglutide injectable medication that I take once a week. It is in a class of drugs known as glucagon-like peptide-1 (GLP-1) agonists (incretin mimetics). This is normally a drug given to people with type 2 diabetes. It does work for some of us with type 1. Thankfully, I am one who has had massive success with this drug.

Since starting Ozempic, my blood sugars stay in range nearly 80 percent of the time, a huge win. Also, the Ozempic helped me lose a bit more than 20 pounds and keep the weight off. Dana noted that my diet was quite good, and that I didn't overeat, yet my weight had creeped up and I struggled to lose even 5 pounds. She suggested Ozempic, and thankfully my health insurance covers me taking this particular medication. One of the key things Ozempic does for me is create satiety. I didn't realize that one of the side effects of my version of type 1 diabetes is that I chronically feel hungry. I almost never feel full. Turns out that causes a low level of overeating nearly every day. The Ozempic makes that constant hungry feeling evaporate, making it much easier to stop eating, and not feel like I'm still hungry.

On the weightlifting front, I hired a personal fitness trainer to help me learn how to use the various machines at the gym I attend. My friend Linda Brandt shared with me a weightlifting program called the SHE program. SHE stands for Strong, Healthy, and Empowered. Linda helped study and implement it with women through the YWCA Minneapolis and the University of Minnesota Twin Cities. It's a flexible weightlifting program that is geared toward women.

The first few times I showed up to work with Erin Reding, the young personal fitness trainer I hired, I was a nervous wreck. Being in a gym with bodybuilders and people who look confident and self-assured easily intimidates me, which has been true for most of my life. Remember the gym memberships I had when I was in my twenties? Luckily, as a middle-aged woman now, I know how to pull confidence into the present moment. I mentioned how intimidated I get, and I asked Erin to help me move around the gym with ease and confidence. We met eight times over the summer. In general, we met once a week and between our workouts, I repeated the workouts she created from the SHE program. Doing what we had done together helped me be more comfortable with the exercises and the machines. The other thing that helped is the SHE program has three parts: (1) four core exercises, (2) nine groups that are nine body parts, and (3) stretching to do after the workout. Each of the nine groups/body parts have beginner, intermediate, and advanced exercises to choose from. This way the program stays interesting, and it allows me to mix things up, so as not to get bored.

I've been weightlifting twice a week for over three years. Slowly and surely a few amazing things have happened in this time. Most noticeable is how much more confident I feel in my body. I walk taller and have better posture. My core is more solid. I move with more grace and ease. I also feel more confident in the gym. I finally feel like I have a right to be there. Another side effect of consistent weightlifting is it contributes to keeping my blood sugars in range. Turns out having more muscle and less fat on the body allows insulin to work more effectively. Confidence and efficiency, a winning combination.

INSPIRATION FROM AN OLDER RUNNER

There's a man named Mike Mann who comes to the track workouts at the YWCA. Mike started running regularly when he was in his early sixties. He's now in his mid-seventites, and he runs much faster than me! So much faster that he recently qualified to run the Boston Marathon. A few weeks before it was held, he ran the Twin Cities 10-mile race, which follows some of the Twin Cities Marathon route. A few of my triathlon friends also did the 10-mile race. I was there watching and celebrating Mike having finished the 10-miles fairly quickly, and his wife, not a runner, was also watching and celebrating the remaining runners. That gave me the chance to chat with Mike and his wife, Vicki. We got onto the role of strength training and aging. Mike mentioned that he does regular strength building workouts. Vicki mentioned that many of their friends and family think Mike is just automatically fast and fit. She said what they don't understand is how focused Mike is on his fitness and well-being. She talked about how careful Mike is to build his strength so that he avoids injury, which is important if one wants to keep running. I love this way of thinking. Mike is a wonderful role model for me. He reminds me of the value of creating lifelong habits of movement and strength.

AGING WITH MOVEMENT

Aging isn't easy for most of us. Our bodies don't heal as fast. We can lose some of our range of motion. Our memory can start to go. It can become very frustrating. I know there are moments I feel like giving up. Then I remind myself how I age is basically up to me. The choices we make on a daily basis will determine or help determine how gracefully aging happens. The things I talk about in this book will help you age with more ease. I breathe deeply and remind myself that as much time I get here on planet Earth is better enjoyed when I make healthy food choices, get enough sleep, spend quality time with friends, and best of all, keep signing up for races and events.

We are who we surround ourselves with, so you might as well surround yourself with people who move their bodies. When we were in high school and college, it was easy to make friends since everyone was going to class, eating lunch, and hanging out. Friendships spring up without effort. Once we get out of school, get jobs, start families, and get dogs and cats, life gets a bit more complicated. Making friends is harder.

The best way that I've discovered for making new friends as an adult is through endurance athletics. When a few of us took cross country ski lessons, we met a number of people that became ski friends. When I joined Run Minnesota and started showing up for the winter Polar Bear Runs, I made many new friends. Consistency and shared activities are the foundation of connection and belonging. Invest in yourself and the people you have around you.

BREATHWORK JOURNEY

I have a story to tell you. In addition to the various jobs I've held, I am a Holotropic Breathwork facilitator. That means that I studied intensively for a five-year period with Stanislov Grof, a psychiatrist, teacher, writer, and one of the founding fathers of Transpersonal Psychology. Holotropic Breathwork is a method of entering an altered state of consciousness using breath and music. "Holotropic" is a word that Stan coined from two Greek words, *holos* and *tropic*. It means "moving toward wholeness." It's a method that Stan developed based on many years of study and experimentation. His intention was to help us access the parts of our brains that are beyond everyday consensus reality. His desire was to offer tools, and a framework, for personal and planetary healing. I found Holotropic Breathwork because I was looking for a way to understand and heal from the deep aloneness, the attachment disorder I carried, and the trauma of the childhood sexual abuse I experienced.

What drew me to Holotropic Breathwork was that it doesn't particularly matter what participants believe about healing or religion. It is a way, without dogma, to have a powerful experience that teaches you about you. One premise of Holotropic Breathwork is that we each have our own Inner Healer. This wise Inner Healer in us is always doing the best it can to help us heal and help us understand who we are. Another premise of this modality is that whatever sort of experience a breathwork session gives the breather, that experience is the perfect experience for that moment in life.

I rarely feel sorry for myself or consider myself a victim of my health or life circumstances. To explain why, I offer you one of the most profound breathwork experiences I had while going through Holotropic Breathwork facilitator training. It's an experience that is a touchstone as I move through my life.

MAP OF MY LIFE

I am lying on the mat in the room filled with fellow breathers and sitters; the loud tribal drumming music pulses through me, awakening my spirit. I know I am safe here in this room of seekers. Gradually, as I breathe the circular breath and ride the music, I feel my mind and body begin to let go, surrendering to this experience. Then suddenly, something shifts and I fully let go. I am no longer in this room.

I find myself in the most beautiful place I have ever known. The air is vibrating with health and vitality. There is an alive energy that is familiar. My essence touches this alive energy. It is so palpable. I walk toward the center of the large open space, and I see before me a stunning, huge, circular three-dimensional map. Like the air, it too is pulsing. I know it's a map, but I don't yet understand what it's a map of, or how I know it is a map. I just know.

At first, I am alone, standing and looking into this map. I watch lights swirl and dodge. The map is alive, vibrating, communicating. It reminds me of when I've been at the planetarium and the show hasn't quite started and they are turning the lights on and off, testing things out. There is shining and blinking and various colors dancing. I feel a deep sense of calm and rightness in being present here. I know I am in the right place. I know that something wonderful is about to happen. Peacefulness flows through my being.

I notice I am no longer alone. Standing with me, all around the map are Beings. They smile at me, reassuring me, sending waves of Love to me. I know these Beings. I am one of them. I ache remembering how close I am to them. There is no separation between us, yet we are distinct. I know that we are here to finalize something that we have created together. This is the last step in the work we have done. We are going to make this map. We have chosen *this* map as *my* map.

Slowly each of them places something with incredible intention into the map. As each object is placed, each Being looks at me, deep into me. I realize the objects we are placing into the map are planets. The map is the Zodiac. As the planets are placed and the geometry comes into view, I realize we are drawing my life, my next human life. There is nothing accidental about the life I am about to enter. There is nothing I will live that I am not a part of choosing for myself. I choose it all because I want to learn. I want this next life of mine to teach me great lessons. In fact, I yearn for the lessons I will have the opportunity to explore. I see that it is the perfect life for me. It is rich with opportunity for growth and development.

I experience, like a wave breaking on the sand again and again, the Love behind the placement of every planet. Each of the Beings encircling the map infuses me and my coming life with Remembering. They do this because we all know that I will forget. Forgetting and falling asleep are part of the exquisite human dilemma. It is part of what makes these lessons so powerful. I *will* wonder, "Why is my life so hard?"

They, and I, want me to spend as little time as possible on this question and instead to spend my human time learning.

They hope that I remember to listen closely to the whispering in my heart and soul that will remind me to know that who I am is much more than the circumstances of my life. And that all the challenges I will experience are gateways to growth and development that my being desires. It will be extremely difficult for me to remember this. Thus for balance, we pour grace, creativity, leadership, inspiration, faith, and yes, athleticism, into the map. If I pay attention, I will be able to draw from these gifts as I face the challenges ahead.

The map room fades, and I am back in my body on the mat in the breathing room again. My face is wet with tears and my body is spent, even though I haven't moved much at all. I know I have seen and touched a truth beyond what I previously imagined possible.

As I reflect on the challenges of my life—the sexual abuse, the diabetes, the multiple rounds of cancer, the attachment disorder, the suicide attempts, the estrangement from my biological family, the challenges I have had with trusting friendships—all of it reminds me that despite these challenges, I chose it. I have learned from all of these horrible experiences. I have survived all of these experiences. I keep searching for and discovering post traumatic growth from these experiences.

Like in that map, when I sit quietly and look closely, my Inner Healer reminds me that I am more than these devastating experiences I have survived. Simply because I exist, I matter, and fundamentally I am whole. I can call on the gifts I have within me to bolster my confidence and my courage to continue on. One of the gifts I call on most often is my inner endurance athlete. She is strong and sure. She comforts me and holds my heart gently and with care.

I offer this story to you because I'm asking you to become an endurance athlete too. Perhaps it's possible that you too have created some or all of the trajectory of this human life before you got here. In any case, you do have choices about how you show up. I encourage you to show up with all the health and well-being you can muster. You are worth it.

AGING AND STAYING ACTIVE

I'm nearing age sixty, and true confession, this age scares me a bit. As we age our bones can become more brittle, many of us develop more body pains, and it's easy to gain unwanted weight. I was talking to a friend, and she went on about her dentures (yes, losing teeth becomes an aging reality for many). That got me thinking, what can I do to help my body as it ages?

Top of the list is to continue consistent, focused movement. Having friends to train with and do events with helps keep me going. Thankfully my knees are holding up well, and while I am not a fast runner, I am a runner. The other thing that I've added is consistent, twice-a-week weightlifting. I go to the gym, and for the times the gym is closed, I have hand weights, a big exercise ball, and a few stretchy bands I can use to maintain my muscles. Luckily, finding a pool for regular swimming is easy. Swimming is very low impact, and I enjoy gliding through the water. I don't yet have an electric bike, but as I age, I imagine I will purchase one, so that I can keep biking all spring, summer, and fall.

I take lots of deep breaths as my anxiety about aging creeps in to scare me. I remind myself to pay attention to what is true right now. Right now, my health is good. I have very little pain, and I am happy with my weight. I then relax and enjoy where I am today. I start planning for my next athletic adventure.

I encourage you too to take a deep breath, sit quietly, and reflect on where you are in your life. Focus on all that is working in your life. Remind yourself how strong and healthy you already are. Congratulate yourself on taking charge of yourself, your life, and your well-being.

TRY THIS

Journal

How are you navigating aging?

Take a moment to write about your feelings about aging. Do you ignore it? Does it bother you? Is there anything reassuring or beneficial about aging? If so, what is it, and can you magnify that in your life? Do you have friends that are dedicated to moving their bodies? If yes, celebrate that. If not, can you imagine meeting some new people and making movement with new people a priority?

Write a Race Report

As you finish up a race/event, take some time to write a Race Report. What went well? What did you learn? What did you eat? How did your gear hold up? Be as detailed as you can be. Remember, you can use this report as you prepare and train for your next event/race.

What's next for you?

Take a moment to think about what you want to do next. What additional adventures can you find? Let yourself pause. Feel the letting go. Then breathe deeply and start thinking about what your next step will be.

Resources

The Swedish Art of Aging Exuberantly: Life Wisdom from Someone Who Will (Probably) Die Before You by Margareta Magnusson, Natascha McElhone, et al.

Forever Young by Mark Hyman, MD

CHAPTER 13

MAKE IT YOURS

"Strength doesn't come from what you
can do. It comes from overcoming the
things you once thought you couldn't."

—*RIKKI ROGERS*

YOU MADE IT.

You've got all the information you need to take the next step to get back in your body and to love your body. You have at least one person who believes in you. (That's me, in case you weren't sure who that was.) The fact that you've picked up this book, read it, and done the journaling prompts at the end of each chapter means you are taking yourself and your health seriously. This tells me that you have the knowledge and the awareness you need to make it yours and make it real.

You have been practicing telling yourself you are an athlete. Belief is where it all begins. Then you explored your health concerns. Gaining insight and awareness of the Stages of Grief (as they relate to your health) and understanding the Stages of Change empowers you to move through the challenges that you face. Having self-awareness and self-compassion as you navigate and adjust your identity puts you in the driver's seat. It allows you to move into becoming an endurance athlete.

Then we explored the fears and obstacles that come in relationship to your health challenges, weight challenges, and your increasing age. In chapter 3, we explored becoming friends with fear, confronting it, and then practicing reframing the fear and obstacles. Learning how to do this will assist you as you begin to go out into the world to get the gear you need and want, and to help you go to the gym or join a cycling or running group. Knowing how to reframe things will bolster your confidence and courage as you sign up for an athletic event or race.

In chapter 4, we dove into motivation. Turns out understanding intrinsic and extrinsic motivation along with inspiration will give you powerful tools as you embrace this new, healthy, athletic lifestyle. Breathe into your new, blooming motivation!

Next, you found a race or event and, fingers crossed, you signed up. That's such a big, important step for making it real. I am so incredibly proud of you. We then explored you being the CEO of Team You. An exciting reframe for how you think about this undertaking. Here we talked about who else is a member of your team. Very few things in life can be accomplished completely on our own. Being human means we are social animals and having supportive, encouraging, engaged people who have similar goals makes all the difference in helping us undertake this new life approach.

In chapters 7 through 11, we dove into some of the critical, nitty-gritty details of gear, nutrition, sleep and recovery, training plans, and race plans. I want you to have deep confidence in what you are undertaking. Good information will make all the difference as you make this big change in your life. Remember, as you move forward in your endurance athletic endeavors, these are five areas you can revisit over and over again. When you're out with your new athlete friends, all are great topics to discuss and share insights. Having a solid base of knowledge promotes belonging.

Then we explored aging and staying engaged beyond one event or race. The idea being to feel the post-race emotions and make plans for what's next. Aging can sneak in and derail us, but we talked about how to give ourselves grace and comfort and keep going.

Here we are! I am celebrating you. I will remind you once again, I believe in you. I'd love to hear from you. Please send an email or message me through social media and tell me what sport you're doing and what race or event you've signed up to do. Tell me how your relationship with your body and your health has shifted.

I'm doing a very joyous happy dance. You're reclaiming your health, your body, your well-being—and that is worth a big fist pump and a high five of love and delight.

Thank you for taking me on your journey. I look forward to seeing you out there moving your body and seeing the light and magic in your eyes.

BONUS CHAPTER

RED RIDERS & RED STRIDERS

"A person who never made a mistake
never tried anything new."

—*ALBERT EINSTEIN*

BIKING IS MY FIRST PASSION. I REMEMBER LEARNING HOW TO bike as a five-year-old and immediately loving the feel of the wind in my hair and my hands on the handle bars. The sense of control I felt over my destiny as I pedaled as fast as I could created a feeling of freedom that I experienced nowhere else in my young life. This connection to biking continued as a teenager and into my adult life, and it has led to my creation of the Red Rider program that's used at American Diabetes Association Tour de Cure events. Connecting biking to celebrating life as a person living with diabetes fit together well in my mind.

Tour de Cure events are fundraising community events that are held in a few cities across the United States. At the start, Tour de Cure was among the premier fundraising efforts made by the American Diabetes Association. At its height, there were more than ninety Tours held in a variety of cities across the United States. During the pandemic, many people who worked with the American Diabetes Association were laid off. As a result, in 2020 and 2021, all the Tours were virtual, and there were only twelve of them.

As is the case with many events, they change over time. I've ridden quite a few of the Tour de Cure rides. For many years, here in the Twin Cities (in Minnesota), more than 2,000 riders participated, along with a few hundred runners and walkers. Participants raise money in a variety of ways. If you raise more than $1,000 you are considered a Champion. I send emails to hundreds of my friends, colleagues, and everyone I know to raise money. I've been a Champion for nearly every Tour I've participated in. It feels good to contribute and fundraise for an organization that does such good in the world for the more than 37.3 million people who live with diabetes in the United States.

Red Riders and Red Striders are cyclists and runners/walkers who have diabetes. Come event day, they wear a cycling jersey or tech T-shirt that says "I thrive with diabetes" across the back. As they're out riding, walking, or running the various distances, others see them and yell, "Go Red Rider!" or "Go Red Strider!"

HOW IT BEGAN

After participating in my first triathlon, I went on to do a number of athletic events that highlighted cancer-surviving participants. I got yellow roses at the finish lines and lots of cheering and love for being out on the course as a cancer survivor. It was an unexpected healing balm for all that I had endured going through the cancer treatments, and it had the same effect on my fellow cancer survivors. I loved being able to identify the other cancer survivors on the course, and I always cheered a bit louder when I was near them. The sense of connection and belonging soared when I saw "my people" out there.

A year after finishing my cancer treatments, I did my tenth Tour de Cure. I'd been doing the ride nearly every year since they began in 1991, having done my first in California well before I considered myself an athlete. At that tenth Tour de Cure, I kept looking around for the other cyclists who had diabetes. I asked about fifty different riders if they had diabetes. One or two said yes, and I was so happy to share that bit of camaraderie. Without asking, there was no way to tell who had diabetes. Many chronic health conditions are unnoticeable from the outside. Except for when I was bald from the chemotherapy, no one can tell by looking at me that I have survived breast cancer and that I've lived more than forty years with diabetes. Yet the difficulty of navigating daily life with diabetes is always on my mind. I think about how much insulin on board I have, if I have enough fast-acting carbs with me should my blood sugar drop, if my pump is full of insulin, if my continuous glucose monitor works today—these are all questions that flit through my mind endlessly all day long.

After doing many athletic events as a cancer-surviving athlete, I wanted and even expected recognition for being an athlete out there riding my bike with diabetes. In my opinion, once the drama of cancer has passed, it's not that difficult to be an athlete. The grind of diabetes, however, never goes away. It's ever-present during all the training and the event. I wanted to celebrate and be celebrated.

When I got off my bike at the end of that tenth Tour de Cure bike ride, I was mad. The new Tour de Cure director of the Colorado office, Sara Prevost, happened to be at the end of the ride asking riders how their experience had gone. Most people were enthusiastic; after all, Colorado is a wonderful place to ride your bike. I was fuming and nearly started yelling at Sara. She took my anger in stride and invited me to join the volunteer organizing committee. I said yes.

Then the work began in earnest. The committee was welcoming, but they had no idea what I was suggesting we do. They thought giving every rider with diabetes a cycling jersey before the ride was impossible. They questioned who would want to identify as someone with diabetes. Having been a high school adviser in charge of spirit wear, I knew that people like to be connected to things that are positive. Identity through clothing and gear is important. I needed to find a cycling apparel company that would design a logo and create a jersey that people would think was cool to wear. The secret to our success would be to create beautiful, welcome energy to the program.

The committee and Sara said OK; I just needed to raise all the money for it myself. I couldn't ask any of the existing sponsors to fund the jerseys nor use any of the committee members to create the program. In addition, I had to make sure I got enough people with diabetes who would be willing to wear the jersey I was going to create. Rather than give up, I chose to use the strength I'd gained moving through cancer to create the program I envisioned.

I recruited my certified diabetes educator and registered dietitian Marcy Robinson and my Team Colorado Wild Women triathlon friend Sandria Barrett to join me on my new subcommittee for the Tour de Cure Colorado. Marcey, Sandria, and I had regular strategy meetings. Marcey was in charge of fundraising. Because she worked in an endocrinology office, she had access to diabetes product representatives who had small budgets for worthy causes. Marcey convinced ten of them to donate to our cause, and, in record time, we had raised more than $10,000 to execute our plan.

RED RIDER SUPERHEROES

Sandria came up with the name Red Riders. We bantered back and forth for weeks about what to call the riders with diabetes. We wanted the cyclists to be the superheroes of the day, the reason all the participants were out there riding. We played with the idea of giving everyone a cape, but, given that we'd be on bicycles, we nixed that one. The trademark color of the American Diabetes Association is red, so we went with that. Then one day, "Red Riders" just came out of Sandria's mouth and we had it.

I went around Denver to as many endocrinology offices as I could, dropping off information about our new Red Rider Program, encouraging people with diabetes to sign up to ride. Slowly and surely, the numbers kept climbing. By the day of the next ride we had 111 Red Riders signed up, declaring they were cyclists with diabetes.

JERSEYS FOR THE WIN

One of my tasks was to find a company to make the jerseys. I am a buy-local kind of person, so I wanted to find a cycling jersey company that was in Colorado. I called the owner of Primal Wear, Dave Edwards, and met with him and his head designer, Tim Baker. They convinced me they could make beautiful jerseys for our event. The Tour wasn't sure how it would work to order jerseys in advance for riders, and how we would hand them out before the ride so the Red Riders would be identifiable the day of the ride. I just kept visualizing and believing it was possible. Marcey and Sandria believed too, as did Sara. Sara had to convince the insider people of the American Diabetes Association, and she did.

I went to a local bike shop and convinced the owner to donate 150 water bottles to our cause. Creating the Red Riders was my full-time hobby. I had a full-time day job, coaching high school principals and teachers, and along the way, I became a high school principal. My full-time hobby of creating the Red Rider Program took another 15 to 20 hours a week. I believed with my whole heart that this program would come to life, so every minute I spent was well worth it.

FIRST RED RIDER RIDE

When the Tour de Cure Colorado ride day arrived, Marcey, Sandria and I, along with the whole volunteer committee, arrived bright and early to the ride start location in Boulder, Colorado. We had all the jerseys ready to hand out. As riders came to pick up their numbers and turn in their liability waivers, we asked if they had diabetes. Those who said yes came over to our table and we personally handed each of them their jersey.

I looked each person in the eye, and I thanked them for their courage to live well with diabetes. I told them, "You are why we ride. You are our superhero today." They went and put on their jersey and then each ride distance departed. I rode the 45-mile route that day and, as I started the ride, I took time to say bye to Sara and Sandria.

As I was getting ready to push off and ride, I asked Sandria if she could figure out a way to read the names of the Red Riders as they crossed the finish line. Sandria, with her DJ background, took on the challenge. She got spotters to go down the road with a walkie-talkie, and she gathered the list of names and numbers of all the Red Riders, announcing just about every single one of the 111 Red Riders as they crossed the finish line.

GO RED RIDER!

Riding the route that day, it made my heart sing to see the Red Riders in their jerseys. Every time I saw a Red Rider I yelled at the top of my lungs, "GO RED RIDER!" I came to realize that "Go Red Rider!" means "I love you, I see your courage, I believe in you. You care about your health and well-being, and I celebrate you." It takes too long to say all that when you're riding your bike, so instead I yelled, "Go Red Rider!"

When I was diagnosed with type 1 diabetes at age sixteen, no one said "Go Red Rider!" to me. I wanted that myself, so instead, I yelled it for others. Offering it to riders as we cycled was a way to put out into the world what I never got. No surprise, but sending that out to others additionally healed me.

We had created such inclusive, joyful energy around the Red Rider program that, in time, the American Diabetes Association national office grew the program to be at all 85 plus Tour de Cure events across the country. These days, more than 15,000 people wear the Red Rider jersey every year. After more than ten years of having the Red Rider program, the American Diabetes Association switched things up, adding runs and walks to the Tour de Cure bike rides but still celebrating people living with the challenge of diabetes for moving their bodies. Then, after the pandemic, the Tour became a backseat fundraising event for the American Diabetes Association.

THE POWER OF BELONGING

Mike Carter was one of my fellow Red Riders at that first Tour de Cure where we debuted the program. Mike had been diagnosed with type 1 diabetes seven years earlier as an adult and was initially in shock about the diagnosis. Doing that Tour de Cure in Colorado and being celebrated as a Red Rider changed his life, he said. Volunteering to help in any way he could, Mike collaborated with me for years, creating the first Team Red in Colorado and helping other Tours create successful Team Reds and Red Rider programs.

What we know is that people crave to belong. In part I know about the desire to belong because for so much of my life, that's what I was looking for. Team Red is a team that welcomes those who have diabetes and their friends, but they don't want to create their own team. Ideally, someone with diabetes captains Team Red and makes a big effort to welcome and coach the team members to raise money and train for the event they plan to do. Mike's passion was making the program accessible to all who needed to be reminded that they were not alone with their diabetes diagnosis.

Mike died unexpectedly, most likely from diabetes complications, in 2017. Learning about Mike's death broke my heart. He was a profoundly generous, compassionate man who welcomed everyone to his circle. Had you met Mike, you would call him your dear friend after one conversation. Mike made a significant contribution to the world of successfully living with diabetes by welcoming everyone he met, raising thousands and thousands of dollars, and contributing hundreds of hours to event organizing. Mike, wherever you are now, know that you were and are loved by me and so many. To this day, just thinking of Mike reminds me to up my volunteering game, and to make sure my heart is open to all who get newly diagnosed with diabetes.

Living with a chronic health condition, no matter what it is, is difficult and a big challenge. Prior to creating the Red Rider Program, I didn't really have good friends who had diabetes; I just knew my dad and my brother, who was also diagnosed. When I got to go to the American Diabetes Association camp for children with diabetes, Camp Needlepoint, as a newly diagnosed teenager, I went as a Counselor in Training, a CIT. The woman who was the Camp Director of Camp Needlepoint was Alex Acker-Halbur. Alex and I became longtime friends as a result of working together at camp for more than three summers.

Attending Camp Needlepoint changed my life because eating meals with others who had to inject insulin before every meal normalized what was not normal in my day-to-day life. I remember joking at our table as everyone tried to guess how many "exchanges" the peaches were in the American Dietetic Diet that we all attempted to follow. The laughter at the absurdity of what we had to do helped me and all the teenagers at the table not feel so weird about the challenge of living successfully with diabetes. These early friendships with other people living with diabetes made me realize how helpful it is to share the day-to-day challenges with others who get it.

It's why the Red Rider and Red Strider programs are so important. In fact, thirty years into the Tour de Cure, some of my best associations are with people I met through the Tour de Cure bike rides I've done all over the United States. Two of those people are Gunnar Nelson and Paul Thorsgaard, who both live and ride bikes here in Minnesota. Both have had type 1 diabetes longer than me, and both of them model excellent health and wellness as they both ride their bikes all year-round, even through the freezing cold and snow of Minnesota. Another dear friend is Tammy McLemore, who I met at a diabetes expo in downtown Minneapolis in 2010. I was riding a bike trainer with a Red Rider cycling jersey in the middle of the expo, talking to whoever would come up and talk to me.

Tammy had just been diagnosed with type 2 diabetes and her mother had died a few years earlier of type 2 diabetes complications. Tammy wanted a different outcome for herself, so she looked around for all the resources she could find. One of the first ones was to get herself to the diabetes expo. She was intrigued seeing me on a bike pedaling away. Tammy loves to meet new people so she came right up to me to see what I was doing. Quickly we were sharing our diabetes stories and talking about how important it is to get regular, consistent exercise. Before too long Tammy had agreed to sign up for the 7-mile route at the next Tour de Cure Minnesota. I promised I would find her. That was the start of one of my deepest friendships. Not too many years after that seven-mile ride, Tammy signed up and completed the 100-mile route at the Tour de Cure.

A few of us trained all winter long to be ready for that ride. We brought our bike trainers over to each other's houses weekend after weekend to ride 3 to 6 hours together to music sets we rotated putting together. Those training days were filled with laughter and so many stories of support and encouragement. I especially remember the Skratch Lab rice bars Helen, Gunnar's wife at the time, made for us one Saturday. They smelled so good as they cooked. Helen insisted we had to pedal another hour before we could have any. The ensuing laughter nearly had us falling off our bike trainers. That year, I broke my ankle, so I couldn't do the 100-mile route, but I did show up to the ride to be there at the end as Molly, and then Tammy crossed the 100-mile finish line. For Tammy, I yelled and rang my cowbell, "GO RED RIDER TAMMY!!"

After the pandemic, the Tour de Cure bike, walk, and run events went virtual for a few years. During this downturn, many of the previous ninety nationwide Tours closed up shop. Organizing a major fundraising bike ride is no easy undertaking. It takes nearly a year of planning, finding sponsors, getting permits for the route, arranging volunteers to staff the event, and food to feed all the participants. Not to mention making sure that all the participants signed up to ride meet the fundraising minimums and are inspired to become champion fundraisers. The pandemic forced the American Diabetes Association to examine its organizational structure and employing tour directors fell by the wayside. I'm grateful that two of the remaining twelve Tours that still happen again in person are in Colorado, where the Red Riders started in 2007, and Minnesota, where I've been involved as a volunteer for many years, along with a team of amazing other volunteers.

POWER OF A TEAM

One of the big reasons I do the Tour de Cure every single year is the power of the team. My friend Paul Thorsgaard, who I mentioned has had type 1 for more than forty-five years and who bikes year-round, is the captain of the team I've joined, Paul's Pedalers. Paul starts emailing us in October and December for the ride that happens in June. He recruits us to join the team, encouraging us to send fundraising emails and, come spring, to get on our bikes and make sure we are riding to be ready for the big event. During the years the ride went virtual, Paul kept emailing us and encouraging us. The first virtual year, I rode 30 miles by myself. The second virtual year, Paul, Paul's brother Todd, Gunnar, and I got out our bikes and together we rode 40 miles to commemorate my forty years of successfully living well with diabetes.

For the few hours we are out on our bikes together, a powerful feeling of belonging and being understood settles over me. My biggest daily health challenge fits in, and I don't have to justify, explain, or teach. Plus I can celebrate all my fellow Red Riders who have on their Red Rider jersey. The lovefest brings me back year after year.

ACKNOWLEDGMENTS

GRATITUDE IS A VERY IMPORTANT EMOTION. IT REMINDS ME to take a deep breath and pay attention to what is going well in my life. I am called to notice the love, joy, and delight that is happening in nearly every moment. Even in the moments that could be construed as difficult.

I am amazed that after nearly twelve years, I've made it to the stage of publishing this book. There are so many people who helped me along the path. You are one of those people, because you are holding this book in your hands. Thank you.

I was doing my seventh YWCA Women's Sprint Triathlon in Minneapolis, Minnesota, in August 2022 and I had a transcendent moment of connection and belonging. I realized as I ran the 5K that possibly for the first time *ever* in my life, I felt connected and whole. I've worked hard in therapy and in my daily meditation practice to get here. This book is the result of finally feeling connected and knowing in my bones that I belong and that I matter. This is true for every single one of us. You too belong and you matter. It is my wish that you too feel this in your very being.

There are so many to thank for finally arriving here. I am naming many people and of course, I will not remember to name many who've been on the journey with me. For all of you, I love you and thank you.

First are my ten beta readers who gave me valuable feedback and affirmed my desire to get this book out in the world. They are Kylea Taylor, who also held many Holotropic Breathwork sessions that I attended and who repeatedly reminded me of my value in the world. Her insightful, wise husband, Jim Schofield, came up with the title for this book. The other beta readers were Jenny Thompson, Kathy Ziegert, Berta Stellick, Nadine Wetzel, Marie Rickmyer, Monica Hynds, Laurie Ladd Goudreault, and Jill Marks. I love all of you and hold you in my heart always.

COACHES

Next are the many athletic coaches who helped me gain confidence in my athletic ability, limited as my talents are in terms of speed or winning age-group categories. In no particular order, big shout-out of appreciation goes to Yoli Casas, Nicole Freedman, Danny Docherty and Run Minnesota, Laurie Ladd Goudreault, Rick Crawford, Celeste St Pierre, Carrie Jackson, and Ginger Vieira.

MEDICAL PROFESSIONALS

Given all the medical challenges I have endured, survived, and continue to navigate, I hold so much heartfelt appreciation for Dr. Rebecca Mattison, Elena Walker, Marcey Robinson, Jenny Smith, Dana Mortenson, Dr. Matt Corcoran, Dr. Jocelin Huang, Dr. Charles Kim, John Falls, Sara Erdman, Sarah Gannett, Whitfield Reaves, Carol LeCroy, and

Dr. Sadie Knickrehm, to name just a few of you who helped along the way.

FELLOW ATHLETES

I wouldn't be here, feeling this healthy and good, if it wasn't for the discovery of belonging with fellow athletes. Close to my heart are all of the women of Team Looking Sharp: Jenny, Monica, Nadine, Sheila, Anne, Marie, Brooke, and Lynn, most of all.

The YWCA Thursday morning runners make 7:00 a.m. intervals exciting. Included are Tom, Mike, Jenne, Siri, Meg, Hilda, Ken, Matt, Matt, Tuyet-Ahn, Caroline, Leah, Nancy, Tim, Kate, Glen, Devon, Jenny, Brooke, Nadine, Nancy, Donella, and many more, I know.

My newest group of athlete friends are all of you in the Run Minnesota spring and fall training programs, plus the wintertime Polar Bear runners. Of particular appreciation: Jenny, Katie, Tanya P, Tanya L, Kathryn, Christy, Marcy, Marise, Colleen, Mark, Don, Howard, Greta, Fast Josh, Tim, Tom, Emily, Kurt, Jenny, Susan, and everyone who makes running fun and super enjoyable.

I live in Minnesota and don't get to Colorado often. Thankfully I'm still connected to many of the athletes of Colorado I met back in my Team CWW days. Especially true through the EnduranceGirls of Colorado Facebook group. Much love to Carla, Joan, Delinda, Ana, Susan, Jeannete, Kay, and Liesl in particular.

I've met so many fellow Red Riders over the years and each one of you has a close place in my heart: Tammy, Gunnar, Paul,

Mike, Don, Ken, Larry Bear, Brooks, Heather, Karen, Scott, Darlene, Diane, Kim, Becky—to name just a few of you.

Special thank you to the many staff people and volunteers who believed in the Red Rider program when I wanted to get it started. Special thanks to Sara, Nicole, Janeece, Tami, Sarah, Marcey, and Sandria.

Along the way, I also want to thank the people who befriended me and rode bikes, swam, and went on runs with me when I had no one else to do these alongside. I especially thank Doug Duguay, Ramsey Shull, Kevin Mastin, and Chris Klebl for believing in my athletic ability when I didn't.

WRITING GROUPS AND WRITING FRIENDS

I've spent countless hours writing alone, yet my best writing was and is done in community with friends. I especially want to thank the Warrior Scribes, Shirlene and Cathy, for meeting weekly through three years of the pandemic. Who knew we'd become such good Zoom users!

I meet every week with my First Book Finish pod: Laura, Pamela, Carol, and Sheri. Thank you for being with me every step of the way. Special shout out to Laura for coming up with the subtitle for this book!

Of particular help was writing coach Rhonda Douglas, who created the program that allowed me to completely finish writing this book after more than ten years of being oh so close.

I meet monthly with my Tribe3 Mastermind: Jody Arthur and Christine Hannon, who I met at the last of Jeff Goins Tribe conferences.

I found Mandala Tree Press because of my longtime, long ago work with the program Link Crew and WEB, where I met the amazing Azul Terronez. Azul and I worked together for at least five years, if not longer. We worked hard, laughed until we couldn't stand up, and created magic for teachers and students so they could transform schools into communities of caring. Azul, his partner Steve, and their team are my collaborators in bringing this book to life. Thank you.

EVERYONE WHO SUPPORTED MY KICKSTARTER PREORDER CAMPAIGN

Turns out writing the book is step one in the process of making a book become real. Step two is getting it published and I needed support to make that happen. Two hundred and one people put their dollars on the line to preorder *Extreme Healing.* Thank you to each of you for believing in me and helping get this book out into the world.

Here are all of your names in love and appreciation:

Monica Hynds, Linda Brandt, Brenda Hanson, Katie McMahon, Jeanine Klotzkin, Martha Arjona Kathryn Bursinger, Ara Rising, Marcy Hokenson, Kathy Ziegert, Linda Saathoff, Susan Keis, Elizabeth Watters, Jenny Thompson, Marie Rickmyer, Sheila Sullivan, Ken Hershbell, Dawn Bina, Christine Hannon, Jennifer Ray, Amy Yonker, Michelle Overtoom, Penny Bell, Maria Linn, Carol A. Stephen, Laura Beeby, Lena Lim, Brooks Benson, Margaret Kelly, Lynn Sojak, Terri Tarbox, Maiya Grath, Jeff Holland, Tracene Marshall, Jill Marks, Andreas Astrom, LaVonne Bluhm, Caroline Sheehan, Colleen Roethke, Danny Docherty, Jules Schlichting-Bader, Emily Quigley, Amber Hanes, Nadine Wetzel, Shirlene Perrin, Margaret Quinnette, Erin Wetherbee, Howard Ojalvo, Karen Kingsley, Kitty Woo Zonneveld, Dixie Le V, Tanya Lundeen,

Shelly MacKenzie, Ramona Carey, Christy Hammerstrom, Jody Arthur, Laura Lynn, Michelle Doerr, Heather Nagy, Heather Nagle, Sarah Hansen, Melinda Vahradian, Lyndsay Gregerson, Kate Varns, Tanya Pokela, Lou Ann Kycek, Mary Gaasch, Pamela Sinclair, Gina Sackman, Deb Kuhns, Melissa Ziegert, Linda Hougham, Anne Parker, Nirupam Chatterjee, Maybelyn Plecic, Rhonda Douglas, Steve Hennessy, Jaime Roberts, Julie McDonough, Kristina Vetter, Susan Ecklund, Rebecca Klopcic Mattison, Paula S. Larson, Jill Pitts, Tami Limberg, Kevin Masten, Andrea Kay Kittelson, Ginger Vieira, Benjamin Prohaska, Melanie Peterson-Nafziger, Sheryl Sandberg, Nancy Lyons, Lindsey Hooker Harjes, Beth Nymeyer, Stephen Ponder, Shelly Kilker, Lauren Bell, Cinta Jimenez, Schyler Manning, Barb Wetzel, Gabrielle Murphy, David Horst, Erin Mandell, Douglas Scalia, Jenne Hongosh, Addie Fowler, Rich Poser, Sarah Lawrence Lupton, Nancy Rowe, Nana Nafornita, Josh Carroll, Kristen Stuenkel, Pam Dellea-Giltner, Susan Engberg, Kelly Tabara, Phil and Laurie Boyte, Celina Pokowski, Carla Kountoupes, Anity Dyer, Linda Harold, Mary Buschette, Youa Lee, Emily Perkins, Cindy White, Amber Kim, Kory Macy, Roberta Brown, Ben Hansen, Lindsey Voorhees, Kathy Ahlers, Carmen Ostermeier, Laura Feile, Sara Newberg, Jolene Kemos, Scott Greenberg, Hal DeLaRosby, LeAnne Stewart, Laurie Ladd Goudreault, Elizabeth Spolyar, Stacey Divone, Cheryl Quick, Gina Brewington, Alexandra Ellison, Angela Past, Mike McEvoy, Michael Grant, Kathryn Rinday, Mark Pinto, Adi, Tim Pratt, David Edelman, Anne Cassia, Michael Flood, R Wes Ridgeway, Tuyet-Ahn Tran, Kitty Shea, Brooke Derrickson, Annie Shull, Susan LeBlanc, Stacey Kreger, Scott and Mia Winter, Kelly Close, Jennifer Larson, Sarah Wiskerchen, Amy Mockoski,

Tammy McLemore, Laurie Scolari, Carla Thompson and Joan Lockwood, Amber Rand, Deb Condo, Kathie Olson, Todd Thorsgaard, Karen Ziegert, Kelsey Baumann, Molly Martin, Sara Prevost, Montana Picard, Michelle Ragland, Alexis Ring, Donella Neuhaus, Kathy Anderson, Micah Jacobson, Tracey Brown, Diane Huis, Amy Anderson, Nadya Sabuwala, Helen Dahlen Lovejoy, Dana Fox, Julie Mott, Sarah Gramlich Howard, Joanie Tepoorten Funderburk, Ken Cole, Don Muchow, Michelle White, Jennifer Smith, Erik Sapp, Manisha Nordine, Katie Cashel, Greta Bee, Colleen Roethke, and Eva Tucker.

READERS OF MY BLOG

I love blogging. Now that the book is out in the world, I am back to regular blogging. Thank you to all the incredible readers who show up and read my blog that I started in 2012. Having you along on the journey reminds me again and again that I am connected and that I have something to offer the world.

FAMILY

I thank my family. Even though we don't talk or see one another, I am who I am because we chose each other before we were born. Thank you for all you gave to me, and for all I've learned as a result of time spent with you. Blessings to you, Mom, Dad, Maureen, and Marty. And to your families, John, Dina, Kiki, Georgia, and Mike. Also, thank you to my grandparents and all my aunts, uncles, and cousins. There were many moments of fun and learning along the path of life.

FRIENDS OF MY HEART

It's taken me an extra-long time to understand the beauty and value of close friendships. I am very appreciative of Ara Rising, Linda Brandt, Tammy McLemore, and Jill Marks for having my back and hanging with me through thick and thin, loss and love.

I recently got another breast cancer diagnosis, and I'm navigating this third cancer challenge using the tools I've outlined and described here in this book. Reflecting it back to me and holding me in their love and light are so many, especially Jenny, Monica, Marie, Nadine, Lynn, Anne, Sheila, and Cathy.

You are the dearest family of my heart.

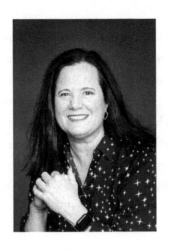

ABOUT MARI

AS A CHILD, MARI RUDDY SURVIVED SEXUAL ABUSE BY FAMILY members and caretakers. She has lived with type 1 diabetes since June 26, 1981, and she has survived three rounds of breast cancer. The trauma of her life resulted in PTSD and two suicide attempts. The theme in her life that allows Mari to live fully and joyfully is her dedication to the endurance sports of cycling, running, and triathlons.

Mari's father was diagnosed with type 1 diabetes when she was one year old; thus Mari has lived with and around diabetes her entire life. She found out she had diabetes when she was sixteen. Her brother was diagnosed with type 1 a few years later. When Mari was thirty-nine, she found out she had breast cancer, for the first time.

Because of Mari's experience being celebrated as an athlete with cancer, she realized the diabetes world needed this, so she got involved as an American Diabetes Association volunteer and created Team Red and the Red Rider Program for cyclists with diabetes, which are now used at all the Tour de Cure events across the United States. In 2015, over 10,000 cyclists with diabetes wore the Red Rider jersey she created. Mari is viewed in the diabetes world as an expert who understands the challenges of becoming an athlete in the face of diabetes and cancer.

Mari was diagnosed with a second round of breast cancer in July 2010. She underwent a unilateral breast amputation with no reconstruction. She gave up meat, dairy, and gluten. Embracing this nutrition lifestyle, with the guidance of several expert registered dietitians, Mari has learned a tremendous amount about nutrition for endurance athletes.

For six years, Mari was the CEO of the company TeamWILD Athletics LLC, training people with diabetes to be endurance athletes. TeamWILD hosted a residential camp for five summers for adults with diabetes to learn how to be endurance athletes. Campers came from all over the globe, including from New Zealand, Australia, and Estonia.

Mari lives in St. Paul, Minnesota, and in addition to her work with the Tour de Cure, she works at the University of Minnesota as an Internship Coordinator. She also consults with a local International Baccalaureate/Montessori high school on internships. Mari loves LinkedIn and has turned that passion into a side gig helping people master the platform for maximum success. Mari has been a high school teacher, a high school principal, and an educational leader and consultant. For seven years, Mari organized an annual event in Minneapolis for survivors of breast cancer to get tattoos over their mastectomy scars for no cost to the survivor. As a result of her varied career and volunteering experience, Mari understands how to explain things in a way that allows people to learn.

Mari is an amateur recreational triathlete, cyclist, and runner. She has participated in more than forty-two triathlons, including a Half Ironman. She has ridden in countless long bicycling events, many at least 100 miles, and running events, including two marathons, so far.

I WOULD APPRECIATE YOUR FEEDBACK ON WHAT
CHAPTERS HELPED YOU MOST AND WHAT YOU
WOULD LIKE TO SEE IN FUTURE BOOKS.

IF YOU ENJOYED THIS BOOK AND FOUND IT HELPFUL,
PLEASE LEAVE A **REVIEW** ON AMAZON.

VISIT ME AT

MARIRUDDY.COM

WHERE YOU CAN SIGN UP FOR EMAIL UPDATES.

THANK YOU!